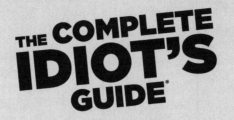

THE **COMPLETE IDIOT'S GUIDE**®

W9-AVX-259

Anti-Inflammation Cookbook

by Elizabeth Vierck and Lucy Beale

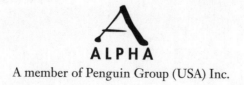

ALPHA

A member of Penguin Group (USA) Inc.

From Betsy: To Jacqueline Schwartz LeClair

From Lucy: To my husband, Patrick Partridge

ALPHA BOOKS

Published by Penguin Group (USA) Inc.

Penguin Group (USA) Inc., 375 Hudson Street, New York, New York 10014, USA • Penguin Group (Canada), 90 Eglinton Avenue East, Suite 700, Toronto, Ontario M4P 2Y3, Canada (a division of Pearson Penguin Canada Inc.) • Penguin Books Ltd., 80 Strand, London WC2R 0RL, England • Penguin Ireland, 25 St. Stephen's Green, Dublin 2, Ireland (a division of Penguin Books Ltd.) • Penguin Group (Australia), 250 Camberwell Road, Camberwell, Victoria 3124, Australia (a division of Pearson Australia Group Pty. Ltd.) • Penguin Books India Pvt. Ltd., 11 Community Centre, Panchsheel Park, New Delhi—110 017, India • Penguin Group (NZ), 67 Apollo Drive, Rosedale, North Shore, Auckland 1311, New Zealand (a division of Pearson New Zealand Ltd.) • Penguin Books (South Africa) (Pty.) Ltd., 24 Sturdee Avenue, Rosebank, Johannesburg 2196, South Africa • Penguin Books Ltd., Registered Offices: 80 Strand, London WC2R 0RL, England

Copyright © 2012 by Elizabeth Vierck and Lucy Beale

International Standard Book Number: 978-1-61564-208-3
Library of Congress Catalog Card Number: 2012933515

14 13   8 7 6 5 4 3 2

Interpretation of the printing code: The rightmost number of the first series of numbers is the year of the book's printing; the rightmost number of the second series of numbers is the number of the book's printing. For example, a printing code of 12-1 shows that the first printing occurred in 2012.

Printed in the United States of America

Note: This publication contains the opinions and ideas of its authors. It is intended to provide helpful and informative material on the subject matter covered. It is sold with the understanding that the authors and publisher are not engaged in rendering professional services in the book. If the reader requires personal assistance or advice, a competent professional should be consulted.

The authors and publisher specifically disclaim any responsibility for any liability, loss, or risk, personal or otherwise, which is incurred as a consequence, directly or indirectly, of the use and application of any of the contents of this book.

Most Alpha books are available at special quantity discounts for bulk purchases for sales promotions, premiums, fund-raising, or educational use. Special books, or book excerpts, can also be created to fit specific needs.

For details, write: Special Markets, Alpha Books, 375 Hudson Street, New York, NY 10014.

Publisher: *Mike Sanders*
Executive Managing Editor: *Billy Fields*
Acquisitions Editor: *Tom Stevens*
Development Editor: *Jennifer Bowles*
Senior Production Editor: *Janette Lynn*
Copy Editor: *Krista Hansing Editorial Services, Inc.*

Cover Designer: *Kurt Owens*
Book Designers: *William Thomas, Rebecca Batchelor*
Indexer: *Tonya Heard*
Layout: *Ayanna Lacey*
Senior Proofreader: *Laura Caddell*

Contents

Appendixes

Introduction

This cookbook offers you answers. Not just the answer to the ongoing question, "What's for dinner?", but the answer to a larger and more serious question. You need to know what to cook for dinner that will help you feel better. You want to lighten your body's inflammation levels. You want to feel at peace about your food selections, without giving up appetizing and satisfying tastes and flavors.

With the recipes in this book, you can do all that and more. You'll find recipes for all times of day: breakfast, lunch, dinner, and snacks. Plus, you'll find recipes for all occasions, from family dinners, to eating alone, to preparing a fancy dinner party for all your friends. Yes, these recipes stand alone as delicious, regardless of the condition of one's health.

Eating simple meals works to sustain life and works well when you're too busy to fix more elaborate fare. Ah, but eating with rich flavors and textures adds gustatory interest to meals and puts smiles of satisfaction on your face. You find both kinds within these pages.

This cookbook offers meals that provide you with clean eating. You'll select organic produce, drug-free meat, organic dairy, and pure cold-expeller pressed oils. You can be confident that the ingredients in each recipe offer you foods that don't increase your body burden of toxic chemicals, as do artificial preservatives, artificial flavorings, artificial colorings, artificial sweeteners, and other mystery ingredients. You'll be eating foods that your body was biologically designed to digest and assimilate for fuel and health.

The recipes give you the means to lower inflammation levels, to lose weight naturally, and to know you're doing what it takes to improve your life, energy levels, and health. Bon appetite!

How This Book Is Organized

The cookbook is divided into four parts:

In **Part 1, All About Inflammation,** we discuss the basics you need to know about inflammation. You'll understand how it originates and learn about its good purpose—to keep you alive—and its harmful side: too much inflammation can lead to serious health concerns and chronic conditions. You'll learn about the body fat connection to inflammation and how to make lifestyle and dietary changes to reduce inflammation. We also review the seven principles of the anti-inflammation diet developed by noted cardiologist Christopher Cannon, MD, and Elizabeth Vierck, co-authors of *The Complete Idiot's Guide to the Anti-Inflammation Diet.*

In **Part 2, Light Meals and Snacks,** you'll discover recipes for breakfast, lunch, snacks, plus soups and stews. They range from easy and quick for everyday "go-to" meals, to fancier fare.

In **Part 3, Main Course Entrées,** expect to find meat, poultry, seafood, and vegetarian recipes. These recipes offer you adequate amounts of complete protein in flavorful combination with vegetables, spices, seasonings, and, occasionally, fruit.

In **Part 4, Side Dishes and Desserts,** expect a rainbow of sweet and savory vegetable and fruit recipes. Other sides include whole-grain pilafs and casseroles. Legumes make eating beans a super treat, with delicious spices, herbs, and nuts. Desserts are yummy while being super health conscious. Have a serving on special occasions.

Extras

We've included sidebars to guide you through the ins and outs of eating the anti-inflammatory way. Here's what to look for:

DEFINITION

With these definitions, you'll learn more about the anti-inflammatory approach to eating.

HEALTHY NOTE

Gain information about how ingredients and cooking methods increase your health.

TABLE TALK

Use these kitchen and cooking tips to make you a master at anti-inflammation cooking.

TAKE CARE

Heed these cautions as you prepare and store foods.

Acknowledgments

Betsy thanks Marilyn Allen for going above and beyond. Thanks to Tom Stevens, fair and firm. And to my husband, Craig, always, always, always. To Lucy: Thanks for making it happen! Thanks to Christopher Canon, MD, for his brilliance in book one.

Lucy gives special thanks to her ever-encouraging and cheerful agent, Marilyn Allen, and to her thoughtful and very helpful editor at Alpha Books, Tom Stevens. Lucy would like to thank her superbly supportive husband, Patrick Partridge, who understands the process of writing and gave emotional and practical support. To Pat, thanks for all the foot rubs and pep talks. To my friend Heather Quinton, thanks for always being just a phone call away, and to her daughter, Tessa Quinton, for her editing assistance. Finally, thanks to Betsy for providing information and encouragement.

Special Thanks to the Technical Reviewer

The Complete Idiot's Guide Anti-Inflammation Cookbook was reviewed by an expert who double-checked the accuracy of what you'll learn here, to help us ensure that this book gives you everything you need to know about anti-inflammation recipes. Special thanks are extended to Rhonda Lerner and Lisa Vislocky, PhD, RD.

Trademarks

All terms mentioned in this book that are known to be or are suspected of being trademarks or service marks have been appropriately capitalized. Alpha Books and Penguin Group (USA) Inc. cannot attest to the accuracy of this information. Use of a term in this book should not be regarded as affecting the validity of any trademark or service mark.

All About Inflammation

Inflammation happens to all of us. Explore how it affects your health—both the positive life-saving aspects and the long-term potentially harmful aspects. The good news is that you don't need to be content living with harmful chronic inflammation. You can do something about it.

You'll learn about the lifestyle factors that contribute to inflammation and how to make often simple changes to achieve a healthier and more joyous lifestyle.

Since the foods you eat play a significant role in ongoing inflammation, in this part, you learn what foods to eat and what foods to avoid. We share guidelines for purchasing food and stocking your pantry. You'll also gain some insight into how foods are produced in our current agricultural system.

Understanding Inflammation

In This Chapter

- Inflammation and your health
- Causes of inflammation
- The inflammation factor in disease
- Ways to protect your health

Inflammation and diet seem to be mentioned everywhere. You've probably read about them in the newspaper, on the internet, and all over the blogosphere. Television commentators and media docs discuss them on the daily news. Some of the information may seem like scare tactics—after all, what could be so worrisome about a diet soda and some chips, for example? The answer is: lots.

As you'll learn in this chapter, having a constant, low-grade level of inflammation appears to be the new "normal." It is a natural response to injury or attack by germs. It can be caused by a poor diet, genetics, a sedentary lifestyle, too much stress, anxiety, or exposure to environmental toxins.

The Inflammatory Response

When you are healthy your body knows how to take care of you and preserve your life, and this is good news. If your body gets an injury such as a paper cut, a scraped knee, or a broken bone, or if you have an infection such as a cold, your immune system rushes to fix things.

The inflammatory response, a key player in our bodies' immune systems, is typically stimulated by some type of injury to the body, even at the cellular level, which involves the movement of blood to the damaged area; delivery of white blood cells to attack any invading microbes; development of swelling, pain, heat, and redness; and loss of function. This type of inflammation is called acute inflammation. It usually appears a few minutes or hours after the injury or infection first occurs. Often these acute responses go away quickly and your body heals.

But sometimes inflammation can be harmful when the immune system erroneously attacks the body. This occurs in autoimmune diseases such as type 1 diabetes and rheumatoid arthritis. These conditions involve chronic inflammation.

Hidden Inflammation

Chronic inflammation often occurs without symptoms. Research suggests that this type of inflammation is the precursor to several conditions such as cancer, Alzheimer's disease, and heart disease. Chronic inflammation is also referred to as whole-body, or systemic, inflammation.

Regardless of our ages, we're all at risk for developing systemic inflammation. However, if you're overweight, your risk increases substantially.

Once triggered, systemic inflammation can go undetected for years while it simultaneously causes irreparable damage to the body. Among the diseases that have been associated with chronic, systemic inflammation are cardiovascular diseases, cancer, stroke, diabetes, age-related macular degeneration, cognitive decline, osteoporosis, and chronic kidney disease.

Many different events and circumstances can cause systemic inflammation including, but not limited to, increasing age; being overweight; eating a diet high in saturated fat (especially for individuals who have diabetes or are overweight), high in trans fat, high in excess calories, or high in omega-6 fatty acids; infections; gum disease; exposure to harmful toxins; elevated blood sugar levels; stress; and lack of sleep.

TAKE CARE

Based on what you have learned so far, if you suspect that you may have systemic inflammation, it's time to start a personal wellness program to reduce the inflammation so that you reduce your risk of eventually developing a serious disease. However, even if you don't think you have systemic inflammation, it won't hurt and will probably help to start a wellness program to avert or delay systemic inflammation.

Unless otherwise noted, from this point forward when we use the term *inflammation* in this book, we are referring to systemic inflammation.

Inflammation and Disease

Mounting evidence suggests that many common chronic diseases are the result of long-term systemic inflammation. High levels of systemic inflammation have these negative results:

- Play a role in heart disease, the top killer of both men and women.

- Contribute to the development of some of the most common cancers, including lymphoma, prostate, ovarian, colorectal, lung, and pancreatic cancer.

- Strongly predict *metabolic syndrome* and type 2 diabetes. In one study, women who had inflamed blood vessels were five times more likely to develop diabetes than other women.

DEFINITION

Metabolic syndrome is characterized by the following: extra weight concentrated around the waist (a 40-inch waist for men, a 35-inch waist for women), blood pressure higher than 130/85 mmHg, a fasting blood sugar higher than 100 mg/dL, triglycerides equal to or higher than 150 mg/dL, and low high-density lipoprotein (HDL) levels (<40 mg/dL for men, <50 mg/dL for women).

- Predispose individuals to neurodegenerative conditions such as dementia, Alzheimer's disease, Parkinson's disease, and fibromyalgia.

- Are a feature of other diseases, such as the numerous forms of arthritis, inflammatory bowel disease, age-related macular degeneration, autoimmune disorders, chronic kidney disease, and conditions ending in "itis," such as pancreatitis.

- Are a factor in asthma, hay fever, allergies, and emphysema.

- Are a factor in skin disorders such as rosacea, eczema, and psoriasis.

Testing for Inflammation

An inexpensive blood test used to assess levels of inflammation in the body is called c-reactive protein (CRP). CRP is produced by the liver. This test measures levels of this protein in the blood. A CRP value higher than normal usually indicates the presence of inflammation throughout the body, without providing specific information about where in the body the inflammation may be occurring. Other tests are needed to determine the cause and location.

A more sensitive CRP test, known as high-sensitivity CRP (hs-CRP) assay is used to determine an individual's risk of heart disease. Studies have shown that elevated CRP comes with an increased risk of a heart attack two to three times and also increase the risk of dying from heart disease. It is also associated with the risk of having multiple heart attacks or strokes.

Your Risk Factors

As previously mentioned, there are many risk factors for developing systemic inflammation. Only one is out of your control—that's your age. To reduce your other risk factors, you need to make healthful lifestyle choices. The following factors affect inflammation in your body:

- Overweight or obese physique
- Age
- Diet
- Smoking
- Sleep
- Gum health
- Stress
- Blood sugar, blood pressure, and triglycerides

Overweight or Obese Physique

Over the years, scientists have discovered that fat tissue is an endocrine organ, storing and secreting multiple hormones and inflammatory molecules and affecting metabolism throughout the body. For example, stomach fat produces high levels of such molecules.

Age

The older you are, often the greater the number of inflammatory molecules you have in your body. The increase occurs even if you're healthy. A number of biological factors work together to cause the increase in these molecules, such as a cumulative dysfunction within cells and life-long exposure to environmental toxins, secondhand smoke, phthalate-containing fragrances, stress, air pollution, and unhealthy foods.

Diet

A diet high in saturated fat increases inflammation in your body, especially if you have diabetes or are overweight. Eating a diet low in inflammation-causing foods appears to be an effective means of preventing inflammation. Several studies published in 2011 and 2012 show that calorie restriction can provide powerful protection against inflammation as well.

Smoking

In addition to causing cancer and emphysema, cigarette smoke contains several components that increase inflammation. At the same time, it reduces production of anti-inflammatory molecules. Smoking also increases the risk of gum disease, which increases inflammation and can lead to heart disease.

Sleep

Sleep concerns, including sleep apnea, insomnia, and other problems that disrupt getting a healthy amount of Z's—about 7 to 8 hours every night—cause an increase in your body's production of proinflammatory molecules.

Gum Health

Your gum health is connected to inflammation. *Periodontal disease*, or gum disease, can produce a systemic inflammatory response that harms heart and kidney functions.

DEFINITION

Periodontal disease is inflammation of the gums around the teeth. This can ultimately result in tooth loss. The newest methods of preventing gum disease are brushing at least twice a day for a full 2 minutes each time with an electric toothbrush; and using a water-flossing machine, such as a Waterpik, once a day, preferably in the evening before bed. If you choose not to use a Waterpik, you should floss twice daily.

Stress

In all its forms—mental, physical, emotional, and spiritual—stress increases inflammation. Stress alerts the body to release the stress hormone, cortisol, which can lead to poor sleep and weight gain.

Blood Sugar, Blood Pressure, and Triglycerides

High blood sugar—over 100 milligrams per deciliter (mg/dL) after fasting—causes inflammatory factors in the blood to surge. A blood pressure reading at or above 130/85 millimeters is on the border of being too high. A tryglyceride measurement of 150 mg/dL or above, as determined by a cholesterol blood test, is a diagnostic criterion of metabolic syndrome, another chronic health concern that is thought to be caused by systemic inflammation. Because each of these factors individually is associated with systemic inflammation, having elevated levels of any of the three measures may suggest the presence of inflammation.

While the preceding discussions about lifestyle choices and effects may sound discouraging, you have the power to make a huge difference in your overall health. You can reduce your inflammation levels by taking positive action steps every day. Later in this chapter we give you specific suggestions to achieve your wellness goals.

Reducing Your Risks

In this cookbook, we guide you in correcting any dietary imbalances you have and set you on a path to delicious—yes, delicious—eating. You'll be averting as much inflammation as you can by eating foods that reduce inflammation and by avoiding foods that increase inflammation.

Anti-Inflammatory Foods

Some foods contain essential fats, known as omega-3s. These essential fatty acids, which must be obtained through the diet because they cannot be synthesized by the body, are known to lower inflammation. They're found in cold-water fish such as salmon, anchovies, and sardines and in flax seeds and walnuts.

Many of our recipes call for these types of ingredients. Simply by eating foods rich in the soothing oils of omega-3s, you can calm systemic inflammation in your body and improve your health.

Low-Glycemic Foods

The glycemic index is a measure of how quickly carbohydrates are digested. Low-glycemic foods are foods with carbohydrates that digest slowly, releasing glucose more gradually into the bloodstream. Examples of low-glycemic index foods include most vegetables, fruits, grains, nuts, legumes, and yams.

Eating foods that are low-glycemic keeps your level of stress hormone, cortisol, lower than when you eat high-glycemic carbohydrates. High-glycemic carbs such as white bread, fluffy white potatoes, rice crackers, and cornflakes are quickly digested, causing a quick and high spike in blood sugar levels.

You can also spike blood sugar levels by eating too many low-glycemic carbohydrates at one time. An example would be eating a huge serving of grains, beans, or fruit at one sitting. When this happens, your insulin levels rise quickly in an effort to lower the blood sugar (glucose) levels, to keep them in a healthy range. These peaks and valleys of blood sugar can lead you to overeat which can, in turn, lead to obesity, which then increases an individual's risk of developing metabolic syndrome, and diabetes.

Low-glycemic diets may decrease blood sugar levels and hence systemic inflammation. Low-glycemic diets also appear to improve blood glucose control in individuals with type 1 and type 2 diabetes.

The glycemic effect of a meal is the overall effect the meal has on your blood sugar levels. Many of our recipes contain condiments that can effectively lower the glycemic impact by one third. These condiments include vinegar and lemon or lime juice, as well as prepared products that contain these ingredients, such as mustards, dill pickles, and some salsas.

Lowering Toxins

Eating more natural foods can help you avoid ingesting toxins that can cause systemic inflammation. For that reason, we recommend that you rinse all of your conventional produce and opt for organic produce if your budget allows. Organic produce typically doesn't contain more nutrients than conventionally grown produce; however, it usually contains fewer, if any, pesticide or fertilizer residues that may be toxic to the body.

You may be able to further this cause by also, if your budget allows, purchasing organic dairy products and drug-free meats, poultry, and fish. Because seafood can contain high levels of mercury opt for chunk light tuna versus solid white albacore. You can purchase mercury-free canned tuna and ask the fishmonger at the grocery store which fresh or frozen fish is mercury free before you purchase.

Eating Good Fats

Our recipes offer you healthy fats (monounsaturated fats and omega-3 fatty acids). We include absolutely no trans fats in the recipes. Instead, you find lean cuts of meat, olive oil, walnut oil, and occasionally a bit of butter for flavor.

We recommend that you reduce the amount of saturated fat you eat from dairy products by using only low-fat or fat-free versions of cheeses, milk, yogurt, and sour cream.

As you cook these recipes and eat the recommended foods in the suggested serving sizes, you may reduce your systemic levels of inflammation, which may, in turn, lower your risk of developing any number of chronic diseases. What wonderful advantages eating well gives you!

The Inflammation/Diet Connection

A convenient way to making reversing or preventing inflammation easy is to follow an anti-inflammatory diet, which provides you with guidelines for what and what not to eat. The good news is that this cookbook provides you with evidence that following the diet can be both health promoting and tasty!

The diet was first described in *The Complete Idiot's Guide to the Anti-Inflammation Diet*. The diet was adapted from the Mediterranean diet, which is a natural inflammation reducer in part because it stays away from the fats that cause inflammation. We include more details about the diet in Chapter 3.

What's Left Out

We know you deserve a treat now and then and that you also don't want to harm your body by indulging in inflammatory foods, so in this cookbook we provide you with some great alternatives that leave out the culprit ingredients but leave in flavor. For example, we admit to loving chips, so we've given you a recipe or two for fries and oven-roasted yams that we think you'll prefer to the ones at the fast-food joints. And we include some yummy dessert options. Only a couple contain sugar or honey; the rest rely on the innate sweetness and luscious taste of natural food. Enjoy!

The Least You Need to Know

- Chronic systemic inflammation appears to be the root cause of many age-related, chronic diseases.
- You can reduce your risk of developing systemic inflammation with lifestyle changes.
- Eating an anti-inflammatory diet can reduce your risk for having systemic inflammation.
- Reducing levels of systemic inflammation may reduce your risk of developing several chronic diseases.

Managing Risk Factors Beyond Diet

In This Chapter

- Identifying lifestyle predictors of inflammation
- Managing body fat percentages
- Reducing stress levels
- Taking action steps for success

It's way too easy to elevate levels of systemic inflammation by participating in a lifestyle that has you burning the candle at both ends. This could mean missing sleep while partying with friends a bit too often; letting stress build up inside you without having an escape valve; shrugging off weight gain because it seems everyone else is gaining weight, too; and eating junk food because it's convenient, cheap, and fast.

All of the above can happen. What's challenging is putting the brakes on an inflammatory lifestyle and doing something about it. But if you're reading this book, we know you're up to the challenge. Others have short-circuited the lifestyle-inflammation machine, and you can, too. Instead of thinking of the changes you'll be making as drastic, think of them as mindful. Think of them as beneficial to not just you, but also your friends, your family, your children, and your world.

Body Fat and Inflammation

A general rule of thumb is that, the higher your body fat percentage, the higher your inflammation levels. They go hand in hand. Researchers have found that being overweight causes inflammation. As if that's not enough, being overweight increases your risk of developing diabetes, heart disease, high blood pressure, high cholesterol, high triglycerides, autoimmune disorders, and other health problems.

This may be tough to hear, but think of it this way: you have one more very important reason to lose weight, if you need to, or to take steps to maintain your ideal weight. You'll reduce your inflammation levels and reduce your long-term risk levels for developing serious health disorders.

Measurement Tools

Using these tools helps you determine whether you're overweight and by how much. They also give you the information you need to set realistic goals for yourself.

First you want to calculate your body mass index (BMI), a commonly used index by physicians, medical health practitioners, and dietitians/nutritionists. All you need to know is your height and weight. The formula (you'll need a calculator) is:

$$(\textit{Weight in pounds} \div [\textit{Height in inches} \times \textit{Height in inches}]) \times 703$$

In other words, divide your weight in pounds by your height in inches squared, and then multiply by 703. If you prefer, you can calculate it on this website from the National Institutes of Health: www.nhlbisupport.com/bmi.

Here's how to interpret your BMI score:

Underweight: BMI below 18.5

Normal: 18.5–24.9

Overweight: 25–29.9

Obese: 30 and above

TAKE CARE

The BMI calculation has some limitations. If you have a highly muscular build, it can overestimate the amount of body fat you have. If you are an older person or have lost muscle tone, it can underestimate your body fat.

If you're within the normal range, congratulations! Your levels of systemic inflammation related to your level of body fat are likely low. If you're overweight or obese, you are at a higher risk of having elevated systemic inflammation levels. It's time to take positive action to lose weight and keep it off. By preparing the recipes in this book, and eating them in the recommended serving sizes, you can lose weight and reach your goal weight.

Body Fat Percentage

To learn even more, have the percentage of your body fat measured. Do this at a health club, at a wellness clinic, or at your health-care practitioner's office. Several methods work for this: the gold standard is underwater weighing, but you'll get reasonably accurate results with a caliper test and with a simple impedance hand-held machine. When you return for a second test, be sure to use the same method as before.

	Women	Men
Essential fat	8–12%	3–5%
Athletes	14–20%	6–13%
Fitness	21–24%	14–17%
"Average"	25–32%	18–24%
Obese	32%+	25%+

Essential fat is the amount of fat a person needs to survive and function well. If a woman's body fat is lower than 8 to 12 percent, for example, she'll stop having periods.

After you have your body fat measured, you can set a goal for the level you want, for most people that's probably somewhere between the fitness level and the average level.

We highly recommend that you use BMI or body fat percentage to measure your success as you lose weight. Stepping on the scale works for some folks, but for others, it becomes a negative emotion machine and it stalls progress.

Managing Your Weight

Losing weight is seldom a cakewalk—it's hard work. It takes determination, relaxation, and mindfulness (being in the moment, purposeful, and non-judgmental), as well as persistence and stamina. And make no mistake—you have your work cut out for you.

You won't find any magic potions, either. So here's what to do:

- Know that others before you have lost weight and kept it off.
- Follow the anti-inflammatory diet, which will help you avoid inflammatory foods.

- Keep your overall goal in focus: to lose weight for health and to look good. Add in any other personal reasons, such as family, job, career, glamour, or relationships. Keep these goals in mind when you eat and when you think about eating.

- Be mindful as you are eating so that you don't just wolf down your food without chewing or tasting. When you eat with true mindfulness, your stomach and senses will be satisfied with less food.

- Avoid trying to keep up with the Joneses, or whoever else you're eating with. The size of your stomach and your dietary needs are different than other people's.

- Be of good cheer. Losing weight takes time. Learn to forgive yourself and to reward yourself with something other than food.

- Reduce stress-induced eating by learning to reduce your stress levels. We discuss this later in this chapter.

- Make regular exercise a joyful and fun part of your life. You'll learn more about exercise choices later in this chapter. Exercise burns calories, but it also reduces stress and lowers inflammation. There's nothing not to love about exercise.

As part of your weight-loss program, you can enlist the support of weight-loss practitioners, personal trainers, and anyone else who can be impartial and helpful.

 TAKE CARE

Unfortunately, weight loss pills and potions have an awful track record. What doesn't kill you either negatively influences your metabolism or compromises your health. The next new pill or prescription may look good or safe, but wait five or six years and always consult a health-care professional before jumping on the bandwagon.

Getting Your Z's

Your body requires a certain amount of sleep every night. The amount a person needs varies based on genetics and other factors, such as age and health. Most folks need seven to eight hours. You can find out how much you need by doing this: for three or four nights, go to bed at the same time and *do not* set an alarm clock. Instead, let yourself wake up naturally. Every morning, record the amount of time you slept. By the third or fourth morning, you'll know how much sleep your body requires.

If, for practical reasons, you need to awaken to an alarm clock, make sure you go to bed early enough to get your required hours of sleep. Yes, this could mean you'll miss the late-night talk shows. But in this case, the price is worth the reward: bright eyes, smoother skin, fewer aches and pains, higher levels of alertness—who wouldn't want those benefits? And your systemic inflammation levels will be lower.

TAKE CARE

Using many cups of caffeine to stay awake after a night of missing sleep is probably fine to do once in a while. But if you use this method often, it leads to a constant rise in cortisol. This breeds ongoing inflammation and can lead to weight gain. Using caffeine can sabotage your weight loss goals.

The inflammation/sleep connection has become better understood in recent years. When you miss sleep, your body's cortisol levels rise. Cortisol is the long-lasting stress hormone that puts your body into fight-or-flight mode. When it's in this mode, your insulin levels rise. That triggers cravings for starchy and sweet foods, adding girth to your waistline.

High levels of insulin predict metabolic syndrome and other stress-related health conditions. The shaky feeling you get the next day is soothed, but not healed, by caffeine in such beverages as coffee, black or green tea, and caffeinated sodas, both diet and sugared.

HEALTHY NOTE

A healthy wake-up ritual involves doing some simple exercises when you awaken. Only 5 or 10 minutes can clear your head and get your energy revved up for the day. You could run in place, do some yoga, or create your own routine of such movements as sit-ups, push-ups, and windmills.

Avoiding Environmental Toxins

Chemicals are everywhere—in the air, in your home, in fragranced household products, in plastic water bottles, in the lining of canned foods, and even in the clothing you purchase. You can't totally avoid exposure, but you can limit it. You can strive to reduce what's known as your *body burden*. Too many lethal chemicals, such as mercury and lead, can poison you. Other chemicals disrupt hormone and endocrine function; still others can lead to cancers. And *all* chemicals increase inflammation.

DEFINITION

Your **body burden** is the total accumulation of all the toxins (i.e., chemicals) stored in your body at a given time. Your body burden may accumulate over the years and can result in elevated systemic inflammation levels. Many toxins pass through the body, but many don't. These chemicals can include mercury, lead, air pollution particulates, secondhand (or firsthand) smoke, bisphenol A (BPA), volatile plastic fumes, and the phthalates in perfumes, nail polish, and fragrances.

You don't need to wear a gas mask or live in a wilderness cave to protect yourself, but you need to be mindful of your exposure. Here's how to take action:

- Trade your old nonstick pans. Better yet, cook in stainless steel or cast iron and expect foods to stick. Using a bit of elbow grease is considered to be exercise, you know.

- Never, never, never microwave in plastic containers or cover the food with plastic wrap. Instead, use glass or porcelain.

- Avoid storing foods in the refrigerator in plastic containers. The chemicals in the plastic may migrate into the food. (A possible exception is dry foods, like cookies.) Avoid drinking from plastic glasses (especially hot liquids). Avoid reusing plastic water bottles, which are actually intended to be used just once. Instead, invest in refillable and safe stainless-steel water bottles to carry with you.

- Rid your home of perfumes and fragrances with the exception of essential oils. This includes perfume, cologne, scented body lotion, fabric softener, dryer sheets, scented candles, room fresheners, laundry detergent, cleaning products, and scented candles. One of the toxins in fragrances is phthalates, which are hormone disruptors. If you enjoy having fragrance around, go natural with essential oils—many smell wonderful.

HEALTHY NOTE

Dryer balls are a terrific and fun alternative to fragranced fabric softener and dryer sheets. You'll save money, too, because the balls last for years. Add two balls to the dryer along with your wet clothes. The balls separate and fluff the clothes while reducing static cling. You can find dryer balls at discount department stores or stores that sell household items.

- Scrutinize your home cleaning products. Most contain harmful and toxic chemicals. Fortunately, some manufacturers offer "green" alternatives, so use those. You can also make your own cleaning products. Mixing up a solution of vinegar and water in a spray bottle is a good place to start. Check the internet for homemade recipes.

- Know what you are wearing on your skin. Read the labels on skin creams, lotions, and makeup. It you can't easily recognize or pronounce the name of an ingredient, chances are good that you don't want to absorb it into your skin. Check online for all-natural skin-care products, many of which are more effective than the "luxurious" brands. Ditto for nail polish, nail polish remover, shampoos, conditioners, and hair-styling products.

- Purchase an air purifier for your bedroom, to remove particulates and volatile organic chemicals, such as plastics, from the air. After all, you spend more time in your bedroom than any other room. You can add additional air purifiers to your home as you desire. Just be sure to clean or replace the filters regularly, just as you do for the air filters on your furnace and air conditioner.

- New clothing, towels, and sheets contain formaldehyde, so be sure to wash them before wearing or using them.

Be sure to stay up-to-date with the news on environmental toxins and take positive action to reduce your body burden.

Stress

Yes, you have stress. We all do. You can't eradicate your stress—in fact, you may not want to. You need stress to get out of bed in the morning, to do your job, and even to have fun. Some stress is good—but too much stress can be bad for the body. You need a balance.

That's why we call it stress management rather than stress removal.

External and internal stress causes an increase in the stress hormone, cortisol. When that happens, levels of systemic inflammation increase. If this continues for an extended period of time where it becomes a lifestyle rather than a blip, systemic inflammation levels may remain elevated in your body, putting you at risk of eventually developing disease.

You can also choose to manage your stress levels which, in turn, can help minimize systemic inflammation levels. Because stress is always present, it's important to find ways to manage it in a healthy way on a day-to-day basis.

Mindfulness

Simply by calming the breath and the mind, you can manage stress. The overall easiest way to do this is with meditation or contemplation techniques: you don't need equipment, and the process is totally free. You can find free instruction for both meditation and contemplation on YouTube and online. You don't need a guru—you just need you.

You can also take advantage of mindfulness techniques through journaling, art, yoga, and other inner, directed activities. Usually mindfulness activities require 15 to 20 minutes once or twice daily. Research has shown that, in addition to reducing cortisol levels, mindfulness techniques sharpen brain function, reduce inflammation, and make a person happier.

Exercise

Believe it or not, exercise can be fun. And fun alone can reduce **inflammation** levels. It takes effort and perseverance to get started with an exercise program, but once you gain some momentum, you'll thank yourself. Why? Because you'll feel so much better.

Current recommendations for the amount of exercise needed to increase health are 30 to 60 minutes of moderate activity a day, most days of the week. Here are some forms of exercise you may enjoy:

- Join a gym and use the aerobic machines, such as the elliptical, treadmill, and stationary bike, along with the strengthening weight machines. Hire a personal trainer to show you the ropes.
- Join an exercise class—Zumba, Pilates, Power Pump, water aerobics, yoga, and more. Make some friends in the class, to keep you motivated to show up.
- Recreate. Go on walks and take hikes. Go snowshoeing or skiing in the winter. Swim or water-ski in warm weather.
- Compete. Play tennis, badminton, racquetball, or squash. Join a group to play basketball or volleyball.

- Purchase some exercise videos, or download routines on your iPad or Kindle and work out in the privacy of your home. You can also purchase a stationary bike or other form of aerobic equipment to use several times a week.

Do what you enjoy to help minimize levels of systemic inflammation in your body. If you have autoimmune disorders or arthritis, exercise is a boon to reducing pain, discomfort, and stiffness. Always consult a health-care professional first before beginning a new exercise program.

Exercise often and exercise well. Everyone you know will thank you for it, including yourself.

The Least You Need to Know

- Altering your lifestyle can alter systemic inflammation levels.
- Get enough sleep to minimize stress.
- Reduce your body burden by avoiding environmental toxins.
- Keep your body fat percentages within a healthy range.
- Use mindfulness techniques to reduce inflammation.
- Exercise for joy and fun while helping minimize inflammation.

Eating for Health

In This Chapter

- The seven principles of the anti-inflammation diet
- What to eat, what not to eat
- True balance in your food intake
- More anti-inflammatory components to add to your diet

Making healthy eating choices to minimize inflammation is challenging, so it's important to keep in mind your end game: a healthier body and mind.

The Seven Principles of the Anti-Inflammation Diet

Your ticket for reversing or preventing inflammation is to follow an anti-inflammatory lifestyle of exercise, weight control, stress reduction, and healthy eating. The anti-inflammation diet is a cornerstone of the lifestyle, providing guidelines for what and what not to eat.

The good news is that this cookbook provides you with evidence that following the diet can be both health promoting and tasty!

The diet was first described in *The Complete Idiot's Guide to the Anti-Inflammation Diet.* Its purpose is to reduce and prevent inflammation and the damage it does to our bodies. The diet is not a program to lose weight; however, because the diet follows sound nutrition principles, if you follow it and also get adequate exercise you *will* lose weight. And that is good news because excess weight is highly inflammatory.

The anti-inflammation diet is adapted from the Mediterranean diet, which is a natural inflammation reducer in part because it stays away from the fats that cause inflammation. All of the recipes in this book are based on the diet, even those that include a dab of butter or a little lean meat for taste.

The point of the anti-inflammation diet is to provide you with a framework to make choosing healthy foods as easy as possible. You will be eating fresh foods that taste great and are great for you! Nothing, absolutely nothing, refined—except on very special occasions. You'll enjoy lean meats in small quantities and butter for flavor, but only for flavor. You'll also be eating lots of inflammation-fighting fish. And your fats will come from olive oil, walnuts, and other good sources.

The diet is straightforward and easy to follow. It has seven basic principles:

1. Eat a well-balanced variety of wholesome foods.

2. Eat only unsaturated fats.

3. Eat one good source of omega-3 fatty acids every day.

4. Eat a lot of whole grains.

5. Eat lean sources of protein.

6. Eat plenty of fruits and vegetables.

7. Eliminate processed and refined foods as much as possible.

The Credibility of the Mediterranean Diet

Many diet plans are on the market promising health and weight loss. Most do not have the strength of research behind them. On the other hand, the Mediterranean diet is a power house of credibility with decades of research behind it.

It all began shortly after World War II with the Seven Countries Study to examine the hypothesis that Mediterranean-eating patterns contributed directly to improved health outcomes. Researchers examined the health of almost 13,000 middle-aged men in the United States, Japan, Italy, Greece, the Netherlands, Finland, and then-Yugoslavia.

Results of the study were definitive. Participants who ate a diet based on fruits and vegetables, grains, beans, and oily fish were far healthier and had less disease than those who ate a typical American diet, which included foods high in bad-for-you fats, sugars, and refined foods. Since that first study a plethora of research has shown the benefits of eating the "Med" way. This list of research results compiled by Oldways is impressive. The diet can:

- Lengthen your life

- Improve brain function

- Defend you from chronic diseases

- Fight certain cancers

- Lower your risk for heart disease, high blood pressure, and elevated "bad" cholesterol levels

- Protect you from diabetes

- Aid your weight loss and management efforts

- Keep away depression

- Safeguard you from Alzheimer's disease

- Ward off Parkinson's disease

- Improve rheumatoid arthritis

- Improve eye health

- Reduce risk of dental disease

- Help you breathe better

- Lead to healthier babies

- Lead to improved fertility

Food and Eating Challenges

As you follow the anti-inflammation diet and enjoy the recipes in this book, you'll learn the best foods and the best food balances for eating healthfully. But the real world can get in your way and derail your plans. Here are some ways to avoid the practical problems you might encounter out there in our food-filled world:

- When eating out, select meals that contain plenty of vegetables and fruits, healthy protein, and mostly low-glycemic sides.

- Pack snacks for road trips and air travel. You never know what kind of food will be available.

TABLE TALK

When traveling, often the hardest food item to find is healthy protein. Pack small prepackaged containers of peanut butter and tuna along with a plastic spoon.

- At a friend's home, you're pretty much stuck with what's served. Ditto for a potluck dinner. If you anticipate problems, eat a healthy snack before you arrive to minimize the amount of food you eat while visiting.

HEALTHY NOTE

When confronted with pizza at an office luncheon meeting, eat the low-inflammatory snacks you keep in your desk for such situations. When preparing pizza at home, replace the crust with portobello mushrooms and the cheese with a 1% version. You'll be in taste heaven.

- Be aware that vending machines and gorgeously packaged cookies, muffins, candy, and cakes can seemingly talk directly to you. They say such things as, "Just this once," "Yes, but I taste so good," or "You deserve a little treat." These are empty promises. Do your best to stay aware of your end game: super health.

- Be polite and kind when friends supply you with treats. Without going into a drawn-out explanation of your anti-inflammatory diet, you can refuse food simply because you don't have anymore room in your tummy or because you're saving room for dinner.

We know you'll be confronted with other opportunities to get off track. As best you can, keep in mind the end game. You may make some poor food choices, but the world won't end—simply eat well at your next meal or snack.

So Many Foods, So Many Choices

In this section, we give you three valuable lists to help you determine which foods to eat often, which foods to avoid, and which ones to eat sparingly. The list is up-to-date as of this writing, but as new foods are created and more research is done on existing foods, the list will change.

Foods to Avoid

The following foods are thought to cause inflammation. Typically, their ingredients have some undesirable characteristics:

- Contain chemicals that may not be good for your body
- Are high in sugar or are high-glycemic, causing spikes in cortisol and insulin
- Contain high-fructose corn syrup
- Contain artificial preservatives, flavorings, or colorings

Inflammatory foods include:

- Foods containing saturated fats or trans fatty acids (partially hydrogenated vegetable oil)
- Artificial sweeteners (sucralose, aspartame, saccharine) and any foods that contain them
- Candy, with the exception of dark chocolate
- Cane juice
- Crackers
- Crisco
- Evaporated cane juice
- French fries
- Fruit juice, unless highly diluted with water
- Frozen yogurt
- "Health" food nutrition bars that contain maltodextrin, soy protein, or sugar
- Ice cream that's not "all natural"
- Maltodextrin
- Margarine with trans fats or hydrogenated vegetable oils
- Meats preserved with nitrates, such as most, but not all, salami, sausage, bacon, and jerky
- MSG (monosodium glutamate)

- Nondairy creamer

- Packaged cookies, muffins, cakes, donuts, pies, and pastries

- Peanut butter that contains more than peanuts and salt and is not labeled "all natural"

- Popcorn with butter, cheese, or artificial flavorings

- Potato chips

- Pretzels

- Rice cakes

- Rice flour

- Sherbet

- Sodas (both diet and regular)

- Sorbet

- Soy protein powder (this is controversial; you may want to discuss it with your doctor or a nutritionist)

- Sugar, including agave nectar

- Sugar-filled sauces, such as barbeque sauce and teriyaki sauce

- Tapioca flour

- Whey protein powder

- White bread

- White potatoes

- Wheat bread, unless it's stone-ground

If you're suspicious of the health value of a food, don't eat it. Most likely, you're right. This includes foods sold in health-food stores and at farmers' markets.

Foods to Eat Sparingly or Avoid

Because they are so easy to overeat/drink and because they can contribute to inflammation in the body, the following foods should be eaten only when serving sizes are strictly followed:

- Alcoholic beverages

- Gluten, as found in wheat, rye, barley, and often oatmeal

- White pasta

- White rice

Foods to Eat

Go ahead and enjoy eating these healthful foods in moderation. We offer you this caution because overeating always creates inflammation, no matter how healthy the food. This section discusses how much to include in your diet in general; in a later section, we talk about how much to eat at each meal.

- Vegetables and fruit

- Oils (olive oil and cold-expeller pressed canola or walnut oils) and monoun-saturated fats

- Nuts and seeds

- Grains

- Seafood

- Meats (low-fat, low-processed) and poultry

- Eggs

- Legumes

- Dairy (low-fat/non-fat)

- Condiments, spices, and herbs

Eat vegetables and fruit often. In fact, eat about three servings at each meal. A good rule of thumb is to have 5 to 10 servings daily. You should be eating 4–5 servings of vegetables and 3–4 servings of fruit daily.

Many vegetables and fruits contain certain vitamins, minerals, phytochemicals, and antioxidants which can reduce oxidative stress that can lead to chronic health issues.

TAKE CARE

To avoid getting "burned out" on eating your vegetables, enjoy the varied tastes of the vegetable recipes offered in this cookbook. Experiment with many differ-ent tastes and textures of vegetables so that you develop a large repertoire of interesting meals and snacks.

Vegetables and fruits offer abundant amounts of fiber, which is important for an anti-inflammatory diet. Soluble fiber in particular helps reduce cholesterol levels. Fiber also increases the transit time of food through your digestive system, allowing less time for substances that are foreign to your body to interact with your body. In addition, in the stomach, fiber slows the absorption of sugars and starches, thus reducing blood sugar spikes.

TABLE TALK

Yams are considered to be healthful vegetables. They are low-glycemic and make a delicious substitute for white potatoes in recipes.

Enjoy oils and fats, but choose healthy monounsaturated fats like olive oil and walnut oil. Make sure your choices are cold-expeller pressed. This insures that the nutritional value of the oil is intact when you eat it. Avoid using oils that are not cold-expeller pressed because they are processed with heat. The heat can ruin the delicate taste of the oil and destroy the valuable nutrients.

Flax seed oil and fish oil contain omega-3 fatty acids, essential fatty acids we need to get from food. Don't cook with these—they don't taste yummy—but you can take them as an important nutritional supplement. By you sprinkling flax seeds on foods and eating cold-water fish such as salmon, sardines, and anchovies, you can consume these healthy precious oils.

Use vegetable oils, such as corn, safflower, soybean, peanut, grapeseed, and cotton-seed, sparingly. Rely mostly on olive and canola oil. The other oils contain high amounts of omega-6 fatty acids; however, when eaten in abundance they can also have inflammatory effects on the body. To reduce inflammation the most, you need to eat more omega-3s and fewer omega-6s.

HEALTHY NOTE

Omega-6 fatty acids are found in vegetable oils, meat, dairy products, and margarine. To reduce inflammation, it's best to eat these sparingly, if at all. Be sure to eat a daily dose of omega-3 fatty acids to keep your body in balance.

For flavor, use olive oil with a touch of sea salt. Use just a small amount to season vegetables and other foods.

Enjoy nuts and seeds in all their many forms. Eat nut butters and add nuts to your salads, vegetables, and meat dishes. Choose from almonds, pecans, macadamias, pistachios, hazelnuts, cashews, peanuts, Brazil nuts, walnuts, and pine nuts. For seeds, use pumpkin, sunflower, sesame, and flax seeds, among others.

Nuts and seeds contain healthy fats and are an important part of an anti-inflammatory diet. For a snack, you can toast nuts and seeds in a skillet or in the microwave and add your choice of spices and seasonings.

HEALTHY NOTE

If you are allergic to a specific food, such as peanuts, dairy, or gluten (even if it is considered an anti-inflammatory food) those foods should be considered inflammatory for your body. You should avoid these foods as well.

Whole grains are low-glycemic and high in fiber. They're higher in calories, though, so be cautious of calories when you eat them. A typical serving size is $\frac{1}{2}$ cup or less. Choose from brown rice, wild rice, barley, wheat berries, steel-cut oats, quinoa, amaranth, and rye.

Salmon, tuna, mackerel, herring, sardines, smelt, shad, and anchovies are good sources of protein and contain omega-3 essential fatty acids. Eat fish several times a week.

Because of the difficulties in our fish supply, such as high mercury levels and concerns about the toxins in farmed fish, it's best to eat wild-caught fish with low or no mercury.

Meats and poultry are important because they are great sources of complete protein. Depending on how they're cooked, these meats can be high or low in fat. However, only 1 to 2 servings should be eaten every week. You need only 3 to 4 ounces per serving, as indicated in the recommended serving sizes in our recipes.

Eggs are a source of complete protein as well. Eat one to two per week, but don't overdo it. Choose free-range eggs, which are high in omega-3 fatty acids, to ensure their anti-inflammatory properties.

Legumes are a terrific low-glycemic, anti-inflammatory food. They're high in fiber and contain protein. They're also high in calories and starch, though, so eat moderate portions, about $\frac{1}{3}$ to $\frac{1}{2}$ cup per serving. You can purchase dry beans and cook them yourself, or take a couple-hour shortcut and purchase them in cans ready to use.

Dairy is high in omega-6 fatty acids, so it's healthiest to eat it sparingly. Hold off on drinking glasses of milk or milkshakes, and limit your intake of cheese. Instead, we recommend that you use dairy as an ingredient in cooking to enhance the flavor and texture of foods. Always purchase organic dairy products from drug-free cows and make sure they are no-fat or low-fat. Be sure to take a calcium supplement if you are limiting the major sources of calcium in your diet.

Spices and herbs hold a storehouse of anti-inflammatory components. Use them liberally. We show you how in our recipes. Be bold, and you'll enjoy the results.

Condiments such as capers, pickles, marinated artichoke hearts, pickled vegetables, sauerkraut, mustard, horseradish, olives, and olive tapenade are healthy for you. Use them often to add yet more health benefits to your already healthful meals.

Some condiments contain sugar, though, so use those sparingly, if at all. These include chutneys, ketchup, salad dressings, and barbeque sauce.

A Balanced Diet

To further reduce inflammation, eat the various components of your meals in a balanced way. At each feeding, you need vegetables/fruit, protein, and fat.

A meal of meat and potatoes with a slice of pie isn't at all balanced. You can modify the meal to contain a chicken breast, a portion of yams, and a salad with olive oil–based or walnut-oil based dressing to create a balanced meal. You can add more anti-inflammatory components by topping the yam with a sprinkling of cinnamon, baking the chicken breast with a topping of walnuts, and tossing the salad with flax seeds.

As you cook, ask yourself what you can add to increase the anti-inflammatory components of the meal.

You can bake a pizza using a portobello mushroom as the crust and using low-fat cheese. Add an apple and a small salad with a walnut oil dressing, and you have a balanced meal that's quite delicious.

The Least You Need to Know

- Manage your food choices based on current research on healthful foods.
- Avoid foods that contain suspected toxins, high-glycemic ingredients, and unpronounceable ingredients.
- Eat 8 to 10 servings of vegetables/fruits daily.
- Herbs and spices contain valuable anti-inflammatory components.
- Eat balanced meals of vegetables/fruit, protein, and fats.

Stocking Your Anti-Inflammation Pantry

In This Chapter

- Refreshing your pantry
- Knowing what foods to toss
- Choosing old-fashioned and simple foods for health
- Going shopping
- Choosing supplements

You know it's time to make a change. Get ready to clear out the old and inflammation-provoking foods and bring in the new. Stock your pantry and refrigerator with the healthiest and tastiest foods available.

Set aside a couple hours to sort through your current stock of food items. Add another hour or so at the grocery store and health-food store to purchase new edibles. If you can't find what you're looking for, don't worry—you can order it online. Now let's get started.

Toss and Clear

The easiest way to clear out space for your new way of anti-inflammation eating is to take everything out of the pantry, the refrigerator, and any other places you store food. Gather a couple boxes or some large trash bags. Wipe down the shelves. Keep a shopping list at hand to add items that you need to replace.

Before you return any items to the shelves, check for the following and throw them out:

- Expiration date—if the food's out-of-date, toss it
- Junk food like chips and cookies
- Rice crackers, white flour, sugary cereal, popcorn, donuts, cookies, baked goods, pastries, and crackers (unless stone ground)
- Sugar-filled syrups and sauces such as chocolate syrup, butterscotch syrup, teriyaki sauce, and barbeque sauce
- Any food that contains partially hydrogenated vegetable oil or trans fat
- Any food that contains aspartame (Equal), sucralose (Splenda), or other artificial sweeteners
- Any food that contains high-fructose corn syrup
- Regular or diet sodas
- Full-fat dairy products
- Deli meats and salads
- Frozen french fries or white potato products
- White potatoes
- Butter substitutes if they contain partially hydrogenated vegetable oils, maltodextrin, or milk products such as casein or whey
- Ice cream that's not "all natural," sorbet, sherbet, and popsicles
- Candy, with the exception of dark chocolate
- Any food you're just not sure of

> **TABLE TALK**
>
> You'll find it easiest to clean out the kitchen by yourself, without loved ones questioning your choices. If your loved ones insist they need their special treats, give them each a small amount of shelf space for their personal cache. While you know that everyone should eat the anti-inflammation way, it's virtually impossible to be the food police for other folks—it's hard enough to do this for yourself.

Restocking the Shelves

Before you set out shopping, make a list. Give yourself plenty of time, as you may need to ask questions and search out special food items. Again, it's easiest to do this by yourself without having to attend to another person's needs.

First of all, the quality of the items you purchase is vitally important. In this case, an apple is not just an apple. Ditto for any other food item. You need to eat *clean*, so pass on anything that contains chemicals that would increase inflammation. As a general rule of thumb, purchase organic, drug-free, free-range, grass-fed, mercury-free, wild caught, and toxin-free foods. These can be tricky to find. Also keep in mind that anti-inflammatory foods will increase your grocery bill.

Bread and Grains

Purchase only stone-ground bread and rolls. The loaf should feel heavy in weight and the ingredient list should be short. If you find dough softeners, caramel coloring, and such, don't buy that brand. Bread keeps well if frozen; it won't stay fresh for more than one or two days if kept at room temperature.

The best breakfast cereals are long-cooking oats and muesli without added sugar. Check labels for granola-type cereals. If they contain sugar, don't buy them.

Choose organic whole grains: barley, steel-cut oats, couscous, brown rice, wild rice, wheat berries, rye, and quinoa. They're often in the health-food section.

Produce: Fruit and Vegetables

Whether you select fresh or frozen produce, try to buy organic. Fresh produce should hold in the refrigerator for a week. Remember, you'll be eating three servings a meal, so stock up on a wide variety of colors and textures.

Some of our recipes call for dried fruit. No-sugar-added and preservative-free dates, raisins, cranberries, and apricots keep indefinitely if stored in air-tight containers.

The Fish Counter

Your best choices with fish are fresh or frozen. Choose cold-water fish that are naturally high in omega-3: salmon, anchovies, smelt, shad, Atlantic bluefish, herring, tuna, mackerel, sardines, turbot, shellfish, and squid or calamari.

Your healthiest choices are fish caught wild that are mercury-free. Ask the fishmonger if you aren't certain.

You can also purchase tuna, anchovies, sardines, and salmon in the canned fish aisle. These are great choices because the fish is caught wild and canned on the fishing boat. Look for the label that reads "mercury-free."

The Meat Counter

Hurrah to the growers of drug-free meats and free-range chickens! They provide meat products that reduce or eliminate toxins in these foods.

Your best choice is grass-fed and drug-free meat. Choose lean cuts, and ask the butcher to trim away any visible fat. If you can't find this healthful meat at the grocery store, you'll find it at the health-food store.

For poultry, choose free-range, drug-free chickens and turkey. For the leanest poultry, select the breast meat and avoid the skin.

Avoid any meat products that contain nitrates, such as salami, bacon, or most deli meats.

Legumes

Purchase legumes in bulk or in packages. Figure that these take an overnight soaking plus two to three hours of cooking time to prepare—except for lentils, which cook faster.

If you favor convenience, purchase canned beans. Rinse them well and then simply add them to the recipe as you would home-cooked beans. You can find them at the grocery store and the health-food store.

Dairy

Purchase only organic dairy, to ensure you that none of the cows that produce the products were fed antibiotics. Choose low-fat or no-fat versions of milk, cheese, sour cream, buttermilk, dry milk, and cottage cheese.

TAKE CARE

To be sure that the produce, dairy, and other products that you purchase are truly organic, look for the seal that reads, "USDA Certified Organic" before you purchase.

Selecting the best yogurt is tricky. You'll find what appears to us as way too many choices. Do not purchase flavored, sweetened, or artificially sweetened yogurt. If you can find plain low-fat organic Greek yogurt, buy it. It has a rich flavor and should contain live and active cultures.

You can purchase regular hard cheeses like Parmesan, Romano, or asiago, because only small amounts are used to add flavor in cooking.

Select organic butter—you'll be using small amounts to add flavor to your meals.

TAKE CARE

Traditionally, yogurt contained abundant amounts of probiotics. These micro-organisms are highly beneficial to your gut health. But as yogurts got fancier, the amounts of probiotics in each container decreased, sometimes to zero. The extra processing, sugar, fruit, and artificial sweeteners destroy these delicate cultures. Avoid the fancy packaging and purchase the traditional cultured Greek yogurt. It's a winner.

Eggs

Eggs are a great source of protein and provide the following nutrients: iron; CLA (conjugated linoleic acid); lutein; vitamins A, D, E, B_2, B_6, and B_{12}; calcium; phosphorus; potassium; and choline. Purchase organic free-range, cage-free, drug-free, all-natural eggs that contain no hormones or antibiotics and have a high amount of omega-3 essential fatty acids. Some brands of eggs are very high in omega-3, with a total of 350 milligrams per egg, with 100 milligrams of the all-important component DHA. Often these eggs contain less cholesterol than conventional eggs.

If you purchase egg whites, check the label. Don't purchase products with additives. The good you do could be erased by the quantity of additives in the container.

The Frozen Food Aisle

Say "yes" to frozen produce, such as green peas, green beans, kernel corn, and mixed vegetables. These are great to have on hand for quick dinners or days when you haven't yet made a grocery store run. You can purchase organic here, too. Because frozen produce is picked fresh and quickly frozen, it often contains more nutrients than when purchased fresh.

Say "yes" to frozen fruit, such as berries and peaches. They are delicious eaten semi frozen and make terrific frostees when processed in the blender or food processor. Be sure you select packages that don't contain sugar or, heaven forbid, artificial sweetener.

If you shop carefully by reading labels, you might find a few gems among the frozen dinners. Some brands offer organic meals with no preservatives or mystery ingredients. If you favor this type of convenience, purchase a few.

Condiments and Spices

Condiments and spices don't only add zest to your meals; they also add important anti-inflammatory nutrients. Here's a list of what to purchase to stock your pantry. Your initial investment could be high, but the good news is that most of these last a long time.

Allspice

Balsamic vinegar—plain and in flavors

Black peppercorns

Caraway seeds

Cider vinegar

Chile powder

Cinnamon

Coriander

Cumin

Curry

Dry mustard

Fennel seeds

Ginger

Low-sodium soy sauce

Mustards—choose plain and exotic flavors

Nutmeg

Red and white wine vinegars

Oregano

Organic lemon juice—found in health-food stores

Poppy seeds

Rosemary

Salsa

Sage

Tarragon

Thyme

Turmeric

Add any other spices, herbs, and seasonings that you enjoy.

Pantry Staples

Keep these items on hand so you can add to recipes for flavor and zest:

Capers	Olives, both black and green
Dill pickles	Organic almond butter
Low-fat mayonnaise	Organic honey
Marinated artichoke hearts	Organic peanut butter
Minced or crushed garlic in a jar	Sun-dried tomatoes
	Unsweetened fruit preserves
Olive oil	Walnut oil

You may also enjoy olive tapenade, artichoke bruscetta topping, and other specialty items.

Beverages

Teas and coffee offer high amounts of anti-inflammatory benefits. They're high in antioxidants and flavonols. Choose organic coffee in either regular or decaf—your choice.

For teas, choose organic white, green, or oolong teas. Herbal teas are especially high in antioxidants, so purchase teas that sound delicious to you.

HEALTHY NOTE

One herbal tea stands out as being the highest in antioxidants: red rooibos tea from South Africa. It's actually bark from the rooibos tree and has a soothing mild, earthy taste. You'll find it in teabags and bulk, and either plain or blended with other flavors.

Adding in Supplements

To ensure that you obtain optimal nutrition, you may need to use some supplements. It's easy to get carried away, though, and think that supplements can provide you with optimal health. You can't view them as a kind of health insurance. And going overboard can be just as detrimental as not getting enough at all.

TAKE CARE

Feeling confident that taking handfuls of supplements will provide you with adequate nutrition is not a valid reason for filling up on junk foods, pastry, and candy. Oftentimes, the isolated food components even found in supplements are not as relevant to the body as those that come from natural foods.

Either in the supplement aisle at the grocery store or at the health-food store, purchase these:

- Fish oil

- Vitamin D_3

- A general multivitamin and mineral supplement, appropriate for your age and gender, containing a USP seal which ensures it dissolves appropriately in your body so that it is usable by the body

- Additional supplements, as advised by your health-care practitioner (physician, registered dietitian, or certified nutritionist)

We prefer fish oil in a lemon-flavored liquid and take a tablespoon once a day after breakfast. In this form, it's easy to digest. If you prefer to take capsules, you need to take three to five daily to obtain an adequate amount.

Some folks who take fish oil capsules find that they burp the taste of fish later in the day. If this is true for you, keep your capsules in the freezer.

Researchers tell us that most folks are low in the vital sunshine vitamin D_3. Sunlight on your skin makes abundant amounts of vitamin D_3. That's great if you live in the tropics, but not so great if you live at higher latitudes. For that reason, take a capsule of vitamin D_3 every day.

Recommendations for how much vitamin D_3 you need vary, so check with your health-care practitioner. Folks with certain health conditions, such as autoimmune disorders, may need more than others. The current recommendation for normally healthy people is to take 600 IU per day.

Low circulating levels of vitamin D_3 are indicated in heart disease, cognitive impairment, asthma, cancer, bone pain, osteoporosis, and autoimmune disorders.

Take a multivitamin and mineral supplement simply because it's a good idea and gives you the minimal amounts you need. You'll obtain plenty of these nutrients when eating the anti-inflammatory way, but a supplement might be necessary in specific situations.

You may want to take additional supplements as advised by your health-care practitioner. These could include additional B vitamins, calcium, magnesium, and others that would aid in any health conditions and optimize your daily health.

The Least You Need to Know

- You'll learn new ways of grocery shopping as you fill your pantry and refrigerator with healthy foods.
- Always purchase organic and drug-free foods when possible.
- Some brands of eggs contain higher amounts of omega-3 essential fatty acids.
- Spices, herbs, and some condiments contain important antioxidants and nutrients that enhance the quality of an anti-inflammatory diet.
- Take fish oil and vitamin D_3 supplements to further decrease inflammation.

Light Meals and Snacks

Preparing healthy and anti-inflammatory breakfasts and lunches was never easier. Cook up delicious meals that stoke your metabolism and help you maintain high energy levels for hours. You'll be eating balanced meals that feed your body and give you confidence that you're taking positive steps to heal your health concerns.

Snacking is becoming a more essential part of our lifestyle landscape. You're busy, and sometimes taking time to sit down for a complete meal conflicts with more pressing things you need to do. You'll find recipes for snacks that you can prepare ahead and pack along with you. You'll also discover some fancier snacks that work well for minimeals and appetizers.

Soups and stews offer light or hearty down-home cooking flavors to appease your appetite and offer you gustatory satisfaction in every bite.

Breakfasts

In This Chapter

- Breakfasts to savor
- Quick-to-prepare inflammation-fighting recipes
- Unique ingredient combinations for great eating

Taking time to eat breakfast stokes your internal anti-inflammation processes. While doing that, you're also stoking your metabolism, lowering the likelihood of gaining weight, and giving yourself a mental boost for the day. You get all this for such a small investment of time.

Unfortunately, although 96 percent of Americans believe that eating a nutritious breakfast is an important part of maintaining a healthy lifestyle, almost one third do not eat a morning meal.

What difference does it make? Well, for starters, people who skip breakfast are more than four times as likely to be obese, compared to individuals who eat breakfast. People who are overweight have a very high risk of developing inflammation-related health problems.

By eating one of the eight delicious anti-inflammatory breakfasts in this chapter (or a similar type breakfast), you'll have higher all-day energy and you'll avoid late afternoon slumps that can lead to binge eating later in the day.

In selecting ingredients for breakfast, choose eggs that are labeled "all natural" with "no hormones or antibiotics." Some eggs now contain high levels of omega-3 essential fatty acids, which contain DHA (docosahexaenoic acid). DHA is an omega-3 fatty acid that sustains normalized brain function, reduces stress, reduces inflammation, and improves immune function. DHA is found in the fatty part of the egg—the yolk, not the white.

Berry-Pomegranate Smoothie

Chock full of vitamin C and antioxidants, this scrumptious, low-fat smoothie is quick and easy to make.

Yield:	Prep time:	Cook time:	Serving size:
1 smoothie	5 minutes	None	12 ounces

Each serving has:				
295 calories	1.6 g total fat	0.9 g saturated fat	5 mg cholesterol	66 mg sodium
65 g carbohydrates	5.2 g fiber	47 g sugars	6.2 g protein	

½ cup mixed berries, fresh or frozen

1 small ripe banana

¾ cup pomegranate juice

⅓ cup low-fat, unsweetened plain yogurt

1. Blend berries and banana in a blender or food processor until smooth. Add juice and yogurt; blend until smooth. Serve immediately.

HEALTHY NOTE

The protein in this smoothie gives you a good start to the day and can recharge your energy in the afternoon when used as a snack.

Overnight Apple Raisin Cinnamon Oatmeal

This tasty recipe elevates oatmeal beyond the merely reliable to a hearty and healthy indulgence.

Yield:	Prep time:	Cook time:	Serving size:
3 cups	10 minutes	8 hours	½ cup

Each serving has:				
185 calories	4.5 g total fat	0.7 g saturated fat	0 mg cholesterol	4 mg sodium
34 g carbohydrates	5.5 g fiber	4.6 g sugars	7 g protein	

1½ cups steel-cut oats	2 tsp. raisins
3 cups water	¼ cup sliced almonds
2 cups apples, peeled and chopped	½ tsp. ground cinnamon

1. Combine oats, water, apples, raisins, almonds, and cinnamon in a slow cooker. Cover; cook on low for 8 hours.

2. Serve warm. You can store leftovers in the refrigerator and reheat for the next morning's breakfast.

TABLE TALK

Put these steel-cut oats on when you go to bed and you'll awaken to their down-home aroma in the morning. Steel-cut oats are an unprocessed whole grain and provide the highest form of nutrition available in oatmeal.

Turkey Sausage and Yam Hash

This version of a beloved comfort food is rich in nutrients and leaves out the greasy spoon.

Yield:	Prep time:	Cook time:	Serving size:
4 cups	10 minutes	13 to 18 minutes	2 cups

Each serving has:				
149 calories	3 g total fat	1 g saturated fat	43 mg cholesterol	53 mg sodium
20.5 g carbohydrates	2.4 g fiber	5 g sugars	18 g protein	

4 oz. turkey Italian sausage, mild or hot

1 small red onion, finely chopped

1 small red bell pepper, cored, seeded, and finely chopped

1 small unpeeled yam, cut into ½-in. cubes

¼ tsp. freshly ground black pepper

⅛ tsp. cumin

¼ tsp. oregano

1. Shape sausage into ½-inch balls. Spray a large skillet with cooking spray.

2. Add sausage to the skillet and cook over medium heat for 3 to 5 minutes or until browned, stirring frequently. Remove sausage and set aside.

3. Spray the skillet again. Add onion, bell pepper, yam, black pepper, cumin, and oregano. Cook, stirring frequently, for 5 to 8 minutes or until sweet potato is almost tender.

4. Add sausage back to the skillet. Cook for 5 minutes without stirring or until hash is lightly browned on bottom. Serve immediately.

TABLE TALK

If you love the taste of sausage, you'll find that this anti-inflammation hash satisfies your taste buds and gives you the health benefits of low cholesterol and low saturated fat.

Stone-Ground Bread with Nut Butter

This quick breakfast gives you all the comforts of a PB&J, but with more nutritional benefits from fragrant nut butters, flax, and 100 percent stone-ground bread.

Yield:	Prep time:	Cook time:	Serving size:
2 slices	5 minutes	3 minutes	1 slice

Each serving has:				
202 calories	9.6 g total fat	1.7 g saturated fat	0 mg cholesterol	203 mg sodium
22.7 g carbohydrates	4 g fiber	6.2 g sugars	8.2 g protein	

2 slices stone-ground whole-wheat bread	1 tsp. flax seeds
2 TB. nut butter (your choice of cashew, almond, macadamia, hazelnut, or peanut butter; see Nut Butter recipe in Chapter 7)	1 tsp. flavored honey, your choice

1. Toast bread in a toaster to desired brownness.

2. Spread 1 tablespoon nut butter on each slice of bread. Sprinkle $\frac{1}{2}$ teaspoon flax seeds on each slice. Drizzle $\frac{1}{2}$ teaspoon honey over the nut butter. Put in the microwave and cook on high for 15 seconds.

3. Serve warm. If nut butter and honey are runny, eat with a fork, or fold over and eat as half a sandwich.

TABLE TALK

Stone-ground breads are available at most grocery stores. Beware of look-alike packages that only pretend to be the real thing.

White Bean Fritters

Fennel gives a slightly sweet, Mediterranean flavor to these savory fritters.

Yield:	Prep time:	Cook time:	Serving size:
24 fritters	45 minutes plus overnight soak time	3½ hours	4 fritters

Each serving has:				
275 calories	4.7 g total fat	0.7 g saturated fat	0 mg cholesterol	275 mg sodium
43.5 g carbohydrates	10.9 g fiber	2.2 g sugars	16.2 g protein	

2 cups white beans, soaked in water overnight	1 white onion, cut into thick slices
3 qt. water	1 TB. fennel seeds
¼ tsp. salt	1 TB. olive oil
	4 TB. black *olive tapenade*

1. Place beans in a very large saucepan with water, salt, onion, and fennel seeds. Bring to a boil, and then reduce heat to a low boil, stirring occasionally.

2. Cook at least 2 to 3 hours so that the white beans become soft. Remove from heat and drain.

3. Preheat oven to 350°F.

4. Mash bean, onion, and fennel seed mixture until the texture of a thick purée. Drop by teaspoonfuls onto a well-oiled cooking sheet, making 24 fritters. Bake for 20 to 30 minutes until lightly browned.

5. Remove from oven and serve hot with black olive tapenade.

TABLE TALK

White beans provide abundant dietary fiber and vegetable protein. If you find them hard to digest, take one of the bean-digestion tablets (such as Bean-O) with your first bite.

DEFINITION

Olive tapenade is a finely chopped or puréed mixture of olive, garlic, and other seasonings. It's tangy and delicious.

Garbanzo Bean Flatbread

Enjoy this crunchy high-protein and high-fiber bread with spreads and snacks.

Yield:	Prep time:	Cook time:	Serving size:
12 flatbreads	10 minutes plus 2 hours or overnight	20 to 30 minutes	2 flatbreads

Each serving has:				
324 calories	22.2 g total fat	2.7 g saturated fat	0 mg cholesterol	105 mg sodium
24.8 g carbohydrates	7.1 g fiber	4 g sugars	8.6 g protein	

2¾ cups water	½ cup extra-virgin olive oil
2 cups garbanzo bean flour	2 TB. sesame seeds or flax seeds
¼ tsp. salt	2 TB. parsley, finely chopped
⅛ tsp. freshly ground black pepper	

1. Put water, flour, salt, and pepper in a large bowl and whisk to blend. Let stand 2 hours or overnight. Stir in olive oil.

2. Preheat oven to 425°F. Lightly oil a 9×13-inch baking dish. Spread garbanzo bean mixture in the pan. Sprinkle with seeds and parsley.

3. Bake for 20 to 30 minutes, until golden brown and crisp around the edges. Cut into 12 pieces. Serve immediately.

Variation: In place of the sesame seeds or flax seeds, substitute 2 tablespoons finely chopped onion.

TABLE TALK

Garbanzo bean flour makes a taste-neutral addition to such foods as cookies, breads, and muffins, lending additional protein and fiber to the recipe.

Omelet with Salmon and Rosemary

Salmon with the fragrant taste of rosemary sparkles in this succulent omelet that's especially high in omega-3.

Yield:	Prep time:	Cook time:	Serving size:
6 wedges	10 minutes	10 minutes	1 wedge

Each serving has:				
155 calories	9.7 g total fat	2.3 g saturated fat	223 mg cholesterol	139 mg sodium
2.5 g carbohydrates	0.5 g fiber	1.7 g sugars	14.5 g protein	

1 TB. olive oil	2 medium tomatoes, seeded and chopped
1 tsp. garlic, minced	3 large eggs
4 oz. cooked salmon, flaked	6 egg whites
2 tsp. fresh rosemary or ½ tsp. dried	

1. Heat ½ tablespoon olive oil in a large, heavy skillet over medium heat. Add garlic and sauté until golden brown.

2. Add salmon, rosemary, and tomato. Cook for 5 minutes, stirring gently. Transfer salmon mixture to a dish.

3. In a large bowl, whisk eggs and egg whites. Add ½ tablespoon olive oil to the skillet over medium heat. Add eggs and cook for 2 to 3 minutes until eggs are set, moving uncooked eggs to sides of the pan to cook.

4. Invert a large round plate onto the skillet. Flip omelet onto the plate. Gently slide omelet back into the skillet and continue cooking. When almost done, top with salmon and garlic mixture. When done, slide omelet onto a large, round serving plate, cut into 6 wedges, and serve immediately.

 HEALTHY NOTE

This recipe uses six egg whites and three whole eggs to lower the cholesterol count.

Quick Breakfast Egg on Polenta

This egg is cooked on whole-grain polenta that's flavored with Italian herbs.

Yield:	Prep time:	Cook time:	Serving size:
1 egg on polenta	2 minutes	6 minutes	1 egg on polenta

Each serving has:				
203 calories	9.7 g total fat	2.2 g saturated fat	212 mg cholesterol	71 mg sodium
20.5 g carbohydrates	0.7 g fiber	0.6 g sugars	8.2 g protein	

1 tsp. olive oil

1 (2-inch) slice Polenta with Italian
   Herbs (recipe in Chapter 12)

1 large egg

1. Heat olive oil in a small skillet over medium heat. Add polenta and cook for 2 minutes on each side, or until polenta starts to brown.

2. Break egg on a small microwavable plate and prick both the yolk and the white with the tines of a fork.

3. Microwave on high for 30 seconds. Open door and stir egg slightly. Microwave for 30 more seconds until egg is barely set. Place egg on polenta. Serve immediately.

Variation: Use a slice of Garbanzo Bean Flatbread (recipe earlier in chapter) in place of the polenta in this recipe.

HEALTHY NOTE

This breakfast takes just minutes, yet offers a high-energy start to your day. Add one or two servings of fruit or a vegetable for a complete meal.

Lunches

In This Chapter

- Preparing healthy lunches
- Incorporating interesting ingredients
- Making dishes high in anti-inflammation value
- Implementing practical options for work and home

Lunch provides a wonderful opportunity to take a break from your busy day and eat foods that actually help you lower the morning's stress and enhance your health.

The ingredients you choose make all the difference in the anti-inflammatory value of your meal.

Choose the following:

- Eggs labeled as "all-natural," with no hormones or antibiotics. If you can find eggs that are high in omega-3, buy them. Omega-3 is found in the fatty part of the egg—the yolk—so be sure to enjoy that part.

- Seek out yams at the grocers—and avoid look-alike sweet potatoes. The yams offer more nutritional value.

- Purchase produce labeled as "organic" when it's available. You'll avoid the environmental toxins found in the pesticides and fertilizers used in conventional agriculture.

- Purchase free-range chicken and drug-free meats.

- Choose low-fat organic dairy products, to avoid added antibiotics and growth hormones.

For this chapter, we've written eight unique and tasty recipes for your lunch.

Yam and Apple Frittata

The unusual combination of ingredients in this flavorful recipe provides a wonderful depth of flavor with a hint of the exotic from grated jicama.

Yield:	Prep time:	Cook time:	Serving size:
1 frittata	15 minutes	35 minutes	$\frac{1}{6}$ frittata

Each serving has:				
175 calories	5.4 g total fat	1.3 g saturated fat	124 mg cholesterol	296 mg sodium
25.2 g carbohydrates	4.5 g fiber	6.2 g sugars	7.5 g protein	

3 tsp. olive oil

$\frac{3}{4}$ lb. yams, peeled and sliced into $\frac{1}{4}$-in.-thick pieces

4 eggs

4 egg whites

2 medium carrots, peeled and grated

2 stalks celery, minced

$\frac{1}{2}$ tsp. salt

$\frac{1}{2}$ cup jicama, peeled and grated

1 large firm Gala or Fuji apple, unpeeled, cored, and thinly sliced

$\frac{1}{2}$ medium white onion, sliced into thin rounds

1. Heat 1 teaspoon oil in a large, heavy skillet over medium-high heat for 1 minute. Add yams in a thin layer so that each slice is touching the pan's surface. Cook yams undisturbed for 5 minutes, then flip each slice and cook another 4 minutes until the edges are brown. Work in batches, placing each round of cooked yams on a plate, and set aside.

2. Meanwhile, break eggs and egg whites into a large bowl, and fluff with a fork, breaking egg yolks. Stir in carrots, celery, and salt. Stir jicama into egg mixture.

3. Add 1 teaspoon oil to the same skillet used to cook yams. Add apple and onion. Reduce heat to medium and cook for 5 minutes, stirring occasionally, until apple and onion slices are nearly translucent.

4. Add yams to egg mixture in the bowl, and then stir in apple and onion slices.

5. Add 1 teaspoon oil to the same skillet, pour in egg mixture, and cover. Cook over medium heat for 15 minutes or until edges brown and begin to pull away from the pan. As frittata is cooking, slip a heat-proof spatula around its sides once or twice and jiggle the pan to make sure it isn't sticking.

6. Remove the pan from the heat, place a large plate over the pan and flip frittata onto the plate. Slide frittata back into the pan (uncooked side down) and cook, uncovered, for 5 minutes. Slide frittata onto a serving plate. Cut into six equal-size pieces and serve.

Variation: For a sweet taste, omit the onion and add 2 teaspoons cinnamon to the egg mixture.

TABLE TALK

Keep jicama from turning brown after it's grated by placing it in a bowl of water. When you're ready to use it, drain and squeeze out the water. Browning is caused by oxidation when the flesh is exposed to the air.

Sesame Omelet with Vegetables

Fresh lemongrass, mint, and toasted sesame seeds add a uniquely Asian taste to this luncheon omelet.

Yield:	Prep time:	Cook time:	Serving size:
8 servings	20 minutes	5-7 minutes	$\frac{1}{8}$ recipe

Each serving has:				
171 calories	11.6 g total fat	2 g saturated fat	93 mg cholesterol	291 mg sodium
8.5 g carbohydrates	3.3 g fiber	4.5 g sugars	8.6 g protein	

4 eggs

8 egg whites

$\frac{1}{2}$ cup chives, coarsely chopped

3 TB. toasted sesame seeds

$\frac{1}{4}$ cup plus $\frac{1}{2}$ tsp. olive oil

$\frac{1}{4}$ cup rice vinegar

1 tsp. sesame oil

$\frac{1}{4}$ cup sweet Thai chili sauce

2 tsp. toasted sesame seeds

8 cups (about 1$\frac{1}{4}$ lb.) cabbage, finely shredded

1 large red bell pepper, sliced thinly

1 large green bell pepper, sliced thinly

1$\frac{1}{2}$ TB. fresh mint, coarsely chopped

1$\frac{1}{2}$ TB. fresh lemongrass, finely chopped

1. Whisk eggs and egg whites in a large bowl with chives and sesame seeds.

2. Add $\frac{1}{2}$ teaspoon olive oil to a large skillet. Pour egg mixture into the skillet and cook over medium heat, tilting the skillet, until omelet is just set, about 5 to 7 minutes.

3. Whisk together rice vinegar, $\frac{1}{4}$ cup olive oil, sesame oil, chili sauce, and sesame seeds in a medium bowl to make dressing.

4. In a large bowl, place cabbage, bell peppers, mint, lemongrass, and dressing. Toss gently to combine. Divide salad among 8 serving plates. Place $\frac{1}{8}$ of omelet on each plate. Serve immediately.

HEALTHY NOTE

The mint gives this recipe a strong anti-inflammatory boost.

Five-Spice Chicken with Broccoli

This aromatic and flavorful chicken dish is delicious served over hot-from-the-pot brown rice.

Yield:	Prep time:	Cook time:	Serving size:
4 servings	20 minutes	8 minutes	1 chicken breast and ¼ vegetables and rice

Each serving has:

344 calories	9.4 g total fat	2 g saturated fat	50 mg cholesterol	111 mg sodium
41.5 g carbohydrates	2.4 g fiber	0.6 g sugars	24 g protein	

2 TB. olive oil	1 TB. fresh gingerroot, grated
1 tsp. garlic, minced	½ cup low-sodium chicken broth
3 green onions, trimmed and sliced	2 cups broccoli, chopped
4 (4-oz.) skinless, boneless chicken breasts, cut into strips	3 cups bean sprouts
1 TB. Chinese five-spice powder	2 cups freshly cooked brown rice

1. Heat olive oil in a large skillet. Add garlic and onions, and stir-fry over medium heat for 1 minute.

2. Add chicken, five-spice powder, gingerroot, and chicken broth, and cook for another 4 minutes. Add broccoli and cook for 2 minutes, and then add bean sprouts and cook for another 1 minute.

3. Remove from heat and serve with freshly cooked brown rice.

TABLE TALK

Be sure to keep the individual serving size of the chicken to 4 ounces. If you can't purchase chicken breasts that are 4 ounces each, purchase a total of 16 ounces and divide equally at serving time.

Chicken Burgers

Ground chicken combined with the slightly smoky flavor of lean Canadian bacon makes a delectable burger.

Yield:	Prep time:	Cook time:	Serving size:
4 burgers	10 minutes	6 minutes	1 burger

Each serving has:				
426 calories	27.6 g total fat	5.5 g saturated fat	111 mg cholesterol	891 mg sodium
4.7 g carbohydrates	1.3 g fiber	0.6 g sugars	39.2 g protein	

1 lb. ground chicken	2 TB. fresh chives, snipped
1 tsp. garlic, minced	¼ tsp. freshly ground black pepper
⅜ cup pine nuts, toasted	8 lean Canadian bacon slices
2 oz. low-fat Gruyère cheese, grated	2 TB. olive oil

1. Place chicken, garlic, pine nuts, cheese, chives, and pepper in a food processor. Using the pulse button, blend mixture together using short, sharp bursts. Scrape mixture out onto a board and shape into 4 equal-size burgers.

2. Wrap each burger with 2 bacon slices, securing in place on each burger with a wooden toothpick.

3. In a large, heavy skillet over medium heat, heat olive oil. Add burgers and cook for 5 to 6 minutes on each side or until thoroughly cooked through. Serve immediately.

HEALTHY NOTE

These chicken burgers taste like they're illegal on this diet. They're a great example of how you can follow an anti-inflammatory diet and enjoy tasty foods at the same time.

Chicken Kabobs

These zingy kabobs are perfect for outdoor grilling or, in bad weather, for baking indoors. Oregano provides an aromatic Mediterranean flair.

Yield:	Prep time:	Cook time:	Serving size:
8 kabobs	15 minutes plus 1 hour marinate time	15 minutes	1 kabob

Each serving has:				
141 calories	5 g total fat	1.6 g saturated fat	53 mg cholesterol	76 mg sodium
3.6 g carbohydrates	0 g fiber	2.8 g sugars	18.7 g protein	

1¼ cups plain low-fat yogurt	4 (4-oz.) skinless, boneless chicken breasts, cut into 1½-in. cubes
2 tsp. garlic, minced	½ tsp. olive oil
2 TB. lemon juice	4 cups shredded romaine lettuce
1 TB. oregano, chopped	Lemon wedges

1. To make marinade, put yogurt, garlic, lemon juice, and oregano in a large bowl and mix well.

2. Add chicken to yogurt marinade and toss well until chicken pieces are coated. Cover and marinate in the refrigerator for about 1 hour. If you are using wooden skewers, soak them in cold water for 30 minutes before use.

3. Preheat the broiler or grill. Oil a broiler pan with olive oil. Thread chicken pieces onto 8 flat metal or wooden kabob skewers, and place on the broiler pan.

4. Cook kabobs under the broiler or on the grill for about 15 minutes, turning and basting with the remaining marinade occasionally until lightly browned and tender.

5. Serve kabobs with shredded lettuce and garnish with lemon wedges.

TABLE TALK

It's important to soak wooden bamboo skewers in water for 30 minutes before using. This prevents them from burning on a grill or under the oven broiler.

Tuna Lemon Wraps

Lemon and cracked pepper add tropical heat to these fun and fast tortillas.

Yield:	Prep time:	Cook time:	Serving size:
8 tortillas	10 minutes	2 minutes	1 tortilla

Each serving has:				
159 calories	7.8 g total fat	1.1 g saturated fat	13 mg cholesterol	168 mg sodium
14 g carbohydrates	2.3 g fiber	1.4 g sugars	8.5 g protein	

8 large (9-in.) corn tortillas	1 TB. lemon juice
½ cup low-fat mayonnaise	1 TB. cracked black pepper
1 (9-oz.) bag (about 4½ cups) spring salad mix	1 (7-oz.) can mercury-free tuna
1 cup tomatoes, finely chopped (about 2 medium)	

1. Microwave tortillas on high, one at a time, for 10 seconds each, to soften.

2. Spread 1 tablespoon of mayonnaise over 1 side of each tortilla.

3. Distribute salad mix and tomatoes equally on tortillas.

4. In a medium bowl, gently mix lemon juice and pepper with tuna. Crumble and spread tuna evenly over tortillas.

5. Roll or fold over to eat.

TABLE TALK

Corn tortillas are a minimally processed grain product made with corn meal, salt, and water. You can make them at home or purchase at the grocery store. Either way, you're eating healthfully.

Quinoa Chicken

Mangoes and quinoa combined with vinegar, raisins, and cucumbers give this chicken dish an exotic, sensational flavor.

Yield:	Prep time:	Cook time:	Serving size:
About 6 cups	10 minutes	20 minutes	1 cup

Each serving has:				
266 calories	7.7 g total fat	1.2 g saturated fat	24 mg cholesterol	76 mg sodium
35.8 g carbohydrates	2.4 g fiber	8.6 g sugars	14.2 g protein	

2¼ cups water

1¼ cups quinoa

2 TB. olive oil

2 TB. white wine vinegar

½ cup mango or nectarines, peeled and coarsely chopped

1 (6-oz.) pkg. (about 1½ cups) cooked refrigerated chicken breast strips, cut into bite-size pieces

½ cup golden or brown raisins

1 cup coarsely chopped, seeded cucumber

⅛ tsp. salt

⅛ tsp. freshly ground black pepper

1 small cucumber, cut into spears, or 12 lettuce leaves

1. In a medium saucepan, bring water to boiling. Stir in quinoa and reduce heat. Cover and simmer for 15 minutes. Remove from heat and let stand, covered, for 5 minutes. Fluff quinoa lightly with a fork.

2. Meanwhile, in a medium bowl, whisk together olive oil and vinegar. Toss with mango or nectarines. Add chicken, raisins, chopped cucumber, and cooked quinoa. Toss to coat.

3. Season to taste with salt and pepper. Serve with cucumber spears or wrap in lettuce leaves.

TABLE TALK

In-season nectarines are a good substitute for mangos. You can also use peaches or papayas to lend a sweet taste to balance the sour of the white wine vinegar.

Fig, Walnut, and Cheese Bruschetta

Three types of cheese are flavored with figs and walnuts for a delicious snack or appetizer.

Yield:	Prep time:	Cook time:	Serving size:
12 bruschettas	30 minutes	None	2 bruschettas

Each serving has:				
360 calories	13.2 g total fat	2.5 g saturated fat	4 mg cholesterol	793 mg sodium
53.1 g carbohydrates	4 g fiber	8.6 g sugars	153.4 g protein	

1 3-oz. pkg. low-fat cream cheese

2 oz. ($\frac{1}{2}$ cup) low-fat provolone cheese, shredded

3 oz. low-fat goat cheese

$\frac{1}{4}$ cup snipped dried figs

1 TB. balsamic vinegar

1 8-oz. whole-wheat baguette

2 TB. olive oil

Dash cayenne pepper

$\frac{1}{2}$ cup chopped walnuts

1. In a medium bowl, let cream cheese, provolone, and goat cheese stand at room temperature for 30 minutes.

2. In a small bowl, combine figs and vinegar, and let stand for 30 minutes.

3. With an electric mixer, beat cheese until well combined; stir in figs.

4. Cut baguette into $\frac{1}{4}$-inch slices. Combine olive oil and cayenne pepper in small bowl; brush on both sides of bread slices. Broil slices 3 to 4 inches from heat for about 2 minutes per side, until toasted.

5. To serve, place toasts in a basket, place cheese mixture in a serving crock, and place walnuts in a small bowl. Let everyone assemble their own bruschetta.

TABLE TALK

This bruschetta makes an excellent light lunch for a picnic or tailgate party. You can add additional finger foods to your presentation: slices of cured ham, green olives stuffed with pimientos, and apple slices.

Snacks and Appetizers

In This Chapter

- Finding snacks that feed your body and health
- Keeping your energy levels high
- Snacking for weight maintenance

Some of us simply need a midday snack or two. While common weight-loss wisdom recommends eating only three times a day, this may not be true for everyone. Snacking is an essential part of health and weight management for many people who want to keep their inflammation levels low.

Provided that you eat snacks only when your stomach is hungry and choose snacks that contain anti-inflammatory properties, you can experience the following benefits:

- Stabilize blood sugar levels in a healthy range
- Continue to reduce inflammation during the entire day
- Increase the amounts of vitamins, minerals, and antioxidants that you obtain daily
- Lessen or eliminate late-afternoon slumps and subsequent overeating

You'll find all these benefits and more in the delicious recipes in this chapter. Be sure to make extras if you'd like to pack some serious snacks for outings, breaks at work, and lunchboxes.

Crispy Calamari

This calamari tastes better than the fried version and offers the flavors of parsley and garlic.

Yield:	Prep time:	Cook time:	Serving size:
4 cups	35 minutes	45 minutes	1 cup

Each serving has:				
237 calories	3.2 g total fat	0.8 g saturated fat	311 mg cholesterol	231 mg sodium
28 g carbohydrates	3.4 g fiber	0.6 g sugars	22.9 g protein	

¾ cup whole-wheat panko	1 egg
¼ cup medium stone-ground cornmeal	1 lb. cleaned squid, tentacles and bodies
½ tsp. garlic powder	2 TB. fresh parsley, chopped
¼ tsp. salt	Lime wedges
⅛ tsp. freshly ground black pepper	

1. Preheat oven to 400°F. Line a rimmed baking sheet with foil and coat thoroughly with cooking spray.

2. In a gallon-size heavy-duty zipper-lock plastic bag, combine panko, cornmeal, garlic powder, salt, and black pepper.

3. In a medium bowl, beat egg. Slice squid bodies into about ½-inch-thick pieces. Including tentacles, pat squid as dry as you can with paper towels.

4. Dip about one quarter of squid pieces in the egg and shake off excess. Add to bag with panko mixture. Seal bag and shake well to coat squid. Spread squid on a prepared baking sheet in a single layer, with pieces touching as little as possible. Repeat steps with remaining squid pieces.

5. Bake for 13 to 15 minutes, until squid is opaque and slightly firm. Transfer to a large serving plate and sprinkle with parsley. Serve immediately with lime wedges.

Variations: Serve with a side dipping sauce, such as tartar sauce, marinara sauce, mayonnaise aioli, or taco sauce. Use this recipe to bake fish and seafood. The results are crispy and fresh-tasting.

Chicken Liver Pate

Enjoy this snack that's very high in vitamins and minerals. You'll find a flavorful blend of onion, garlic, bay leaf, and rosemary blended with chicken livers and cream cheese.

Yield:	Prep time:	Cook time:	Serving size:
About 2 cups	15 minutes	10 to 13 minutes	⅓ cup

Each serving has:				
95 calories	4.1 g total fat	1.4 g saturated fat	216 mg cholesterol	208 mg sodium
2.6 mg carbohydrates	0 g fiber	0.6 g sugars	11.5 g protein	

1 tsp. butter	½ lb. chicken livers, washed and trimmed
1 tsp. olive oil	¼ tsp. salt
1 small red onion, chopped	¼ tsp. freshly ground black pepper
1 tsp. garlic, minced	3 oz. fat-free cream cheese
1 bay leaf	
1 tsp. dried rosemary, crushed	

1. Heat butter and olive oil in a nonstick skillet. Add onion, garlic, bay leaf, and rosemary. Cook over medium heat, stirring occasionally, for about 5 minutes until softened.

2. Add chicken livers to the skillet and cook for 5 to 8 minutes until cooked and no longer pink. Remove bay leaf and let cool for 10 minutes.

3. Place chicken liver mixture in a blender or food processor with salt, pepper, and cream cheese. Purée until smooth. Transfer to a serving dish, cover, and chill for at least 2 hours.

4. Serve with salad or vegetable scoopers. Store in an airtight container in the refrigerator for up to 3 days.

TABLE TALK

For serving, use vegetable scoopers such as celery stalks, carrot sticks, jicama rounds, radishes, or cucumber rounds. These add fiber, taste, and more antioxidants to your snack.

Chicken Tarragon Pinwheels

Tarragon gives chicken a bright, light, peppery-herbal flavor that's hard to resist in these creative pinwheels.

Yield:	Prep time:	Cook time:	Serving size:
2 chicken breasts	15 minutes	10 to 12 minutes	½ chicken breast

Each serving has:				
143 calories	6.6 g total fat	1.4 g saturated fat	40 mg cholesterol	193 mg sodium
3.5 g carbohydrates	0 g fiber	0 g sugars	17.4 g protein	

2 TB. pine nuts, lightly toasted	3 oz. low-fat cream cheese, softened to room temperature
2 TB. fresh parsley, chopped	4 leaves Bibb lettuce
2 TB. fresh tarragon, chopped	1 lemon, cut into 4 wedges
1 tsp. garlic, minced	Parsley sprigs
1 TB. lemon zest, grated	
2 large boneless, skinless chicken breasts	

1. Place pine nuts into a food processor with the parsley, tarragon, garlic, and lemon zest. Pulse several times to purée.

2. Pound chicken breasts lightly to flatten them. Spread them on one side with cream cheese and top with pine nut mixture. Roll them up from one short end to the other so that filling is enclosed. Wrap rolls individually in aluminum foil and seal well. Transfer to a steamer or a metal colander placed over a pan of boiling water. Cover tightly and steam for 10 to 12 minutes or until cooked through.

3. Arrange lettuce leaves on a large serving platter. Remove chicken from heat, discard the foil, and cut chicken rolls into slices. Arrange chicken slices on salad leaves, and garnish with lemon wedges and parsley sprigs.

TABLE TALK

You can also grill the pinwheels over medium coals or bake at 350°F for about 20 minutes.

Thai Chicken Kabobs

Traditional Thai flavorings of sesame oil and sweet chili sauce lend authentic flavor to these kabobs.

Yield:	Prep time:	Cook time:	Serving size:
8 kabobs	10 minutes plus 1 hour marinate time	12 minutes	2 kabobs

Each serving has:				
221 calories	15 g total fat	2 g saturated fat	25 mg cholesterol	191 mg sodium
8.6 g carbohydrates	2.1 g fiber	3.2 g sugars	14.1 g protein	

1 TB. olive oil	⅓ cup crunchy all-natural peanut butter
1 TB. sesame oil	1½ TB. Thai sweet chili sauce
4 TB. lime juice	6 to 8 TB. water
2 (6-oz.) boneless, skinless chicken breasts, cut into 1-in. cubes	

1. Combine olive oil, sesame oil, and 2 tablespoons lime juice in a medium non-metallic dish. Add chicken, cover, and marinate for 1 hour. Soak 8 wooden skewers in cold water for 30 minutes before use, to prevent burning.

2. In a heavy skillet over low heat, stir peanut butter to soften. Stir in chili sauce, water, and 2 tablespoons lime juice, and cook until all ingredients are warm, about 2 minutes.

3. Meanwhile, drain chicken cubes and thread onto the wooden skewers. Put under a hot broiler or on a barbeque, turning frequently, for about 10 minutes, until cooked and browned. Serve hot with the warm peanut butter dip.

TABLE TALK

If you prefer a hotter taste, add more Thai chili sauce. If you like it milder, use less.

Paprika Walnuts

Paprika gives a snappy taste to these toasted omega-3-rich walnuts.

Yield:	Prep time:	Cook time:	Serving size:
2 cups	5 minutes	5 to 7 minutes	¼ cup

Each serving has:				
211 calories	19.8 g total fat	1.2 g saturated fat	0 mg cholesterol	149 mg sodium
4.8 g carbohydrates	2.8 g fiber	1.1 g sugars	7.8 g protein	

2 TB. paprika	½ tsp. salt
1 tsp. freshly ground black pepper	2 tsp. olive oil
1 tsp. sugar	2 cups walnuts
½ tsp. ground coriander	

1. In a small bowl, stir together paprika, pepper, sugar, coriander, and salt.

2. In a large skillet, heat oil over medium heat. Add nuts and toss until well coated. Gradually sprinkle paprika mixture over nuts, stirring to combine. Continue cooking and stirring for 3 to 5 minutes until mixture is fragrant and walnuts are lightly toasted.

3. Remove from heat, cool, and store in an airtight container. Can be stored for 3 months.

TABLE TALK

These walnuts are very high in good fats—the omega-3 essential fatty acids. Snacking on them is a superb way to lower inflammation and enjoy their delicious taste.

Rosemary Roasted Chickpeas

Rosemary and garlic give these crunchy legumes a wonderful taste and aroma.

Yield:	Prep time:	Cook time:	Serving size:
1½ cups	5 minutes	35 minutes plus cool time	¼ cup

Each serving has:				
279 calories	6.6 g total fat	0.8 g saturated fat	0 mg cholesterol	114 mg sodium
43.3 g carbohydrates	12.5 g fiber	7.7 g sugars	13.8 g protein	

1 can (15-oz.) chickpeas, drained, rinsed, and patted dry	1 tsp. dried rosemary, crushed
1 TB. olive oil	¼ tsp. garlic powder
	¼ tsp. salt

1. Preheat oven to 400°F. In a medium bowl, toss chickpeas with oil, rosemary, garlic powder, and salt. Spread on a rimmed baking sheet.

2. Roast for 35 minutes, shaking the pan twice during baking, until chickpeas are crisp and dry. Turn off the oven, but don't remove chickpeas until they are cool. Store in an airtight container for up to 3 months.

TABLE TALK

Enjoy this high-powered protein snack between meals or to lend an added crunch to your dinner salad.

Flax Seed and Oat Crackers

The crisp and crunchy texture of these crackers offers a bit of sweetness and an all-natural grain taste.

Yield:	Prep time:	Cook time:	Serving size:
4 dozen crackers	15 minutes	12 to 15 minutes	4 crackers

Each serving has:				
142 calories	8.1 g total fat	1.1 g saturated fat	0 mg cholesterol	61 mg sodium
14.8 g carbohydrates	1.5 g fiber	1.8 g sugars	2.5 g protein	

³⁄₄ cup old-fashioned rolled oats	¼ tsp. salt
1 cup stone-ground flour	¼ cup plus 2 TB. olive oil
½ cup oat bran	1 TB. honey
3 TB. flax seeds	½ cup water

1. Preheat the oven to 350°F. Lightly oil a large baking sheet.

2. In a food processor, process oats to a fine meal. In a medium bowl, whisk together oatmeal, flour, bran, flax seeds, and salt.

3. In a large bowl, blend together oil and honey. Stir in flour mixture and water, and then mix just until dough is smooth.

4. Press or roll dough to a ¹⁄₈-inch thickness right on the baking sheet. With a sharp knife, cut dough into 2-inch squares.

5. Bake for 12 to 15 minutes or until lightly golden. Cool. Remove from the baking sheet and store in an airtight container for up to 3 months.

HEALTHY NOTE

Use these as you would any cracker. But they aren't just any cracker—you'll be enjoying the superb omerga-3 essential fatty acids in the flax seeds.

Artichoke Spinach Dip

Artichokes and spinach blend perfectly with low-fat cheese and Parmesan.

Yield:	Prep time:	Cook time:	Serving size:
About 4 cups	5 minutes	20 to 25 minutes	½ cup

Each serving has:				
142 calories	10.1 g total fat	2.3 g saturated fat	15 mg cholesterol	433 mg sodium
5 g carbohydrates	1.5 g fiber	1.2 g sugars	6.2 g protein	

1 (10-oz.) package frozen spinach, thawed, squeezed dry, and chopped	½ cup freshly grated Parmesan
1 (6-oz.) can artichoke hearts, thinly sliced and patted dry	¾ cup low-fat mayonnaise
½ cup (4-oz.) low-fat mozzarella, shredded	¾ cup no-fat sour cream

1. Preheat the oven to 425°F.

2. In a large bowl, mix spinach, artichoke hearts, mozzarella, ¼ cup Parmesan, mayonnaise, and sour cream. Transfer to a 1-quart baking dish and sprinkle with remaining ¼ cup Parmesan.

3. Bake 20 to 25 minutes until slightly browned. Let cool slightly and serve.

TABLE TALK

Place the baking rack in the middle of the oven, to get equal heating at the top and bottom of the dip and ensure that the dip will be warm throughout. Serve with vegetable scoopers such as bell peppers, celery, and carrots.

Sesame Almond Squares

Raw seeds, dried fruit, and nuts combine for a high-energy snack that tastes great.

Yield:	Prep time:	Cook time:	Serving size:
64 pieces	10 minutes plus 4 hours refrigeration time	None	1 piece

Each serving has:				
32 calories	1.9 g total fat	0 g saturated fat	0 mg cholesterol	10 mg sodium
3.3 g carbohydrates	0.5 g fiber	2.2 g sugars	1.1 g protein	

¼ cup honey

⅓ cup almond butter

¾ cup nonfat dry milk

½ cup oat bran

½ cup sesame seeds

¼ cup flax seeds

¼ cup raisins

¼ cup unsweetened shredded coconut

1. In a large bowl, combine honey, almond butter, dry milk, oat bran, sesame seeds, flax seeds, raisins, and coconut.

2. Spread mixture into an 8×8-inch baking pan and refrigerate for 4 hours. Cut into 1-inch squares. Store in an airtight container for up to 3 months.

HEALTHY NOTE

Enjoy one piece of these high-energy squares when you need a quick lift, or enjoy with a soothing afternoon cup of tea.

Sun-Dried Tomato Hummus

Middle Eastern hummus is combined with sun-dried tomatoes to give a slightly sweet accent along with garlic and lemon juice.

Yield:	Prep time:	Cook time:	Serving size:
1¼ cups	10 minutes	None	3 tablespoons

Each serving has:				
144 calories	6.2 g total fat	0.5 g saturated fat	4 mg cholesterol	451 mg sodium
17.1 g carbohydrates	3.1 g fiber	0 g sugars	3.5 g protein	

1 can (15-oz.) garbanzo beans or chickpeas, rinsed and drained	1 TB. sun-dried tomato paste
⅓ cup low-fat mayonnaise	½ tsp. garlic, minced
	1 tsp. lemon juice

1. In a food processor or blender, combine beans or chickpeas, mayonnaise, tomato paste, garlic, and lemon juice. Process until smooth. Transfer to a small serving bowl. Store in an airtight container in the refrigerator for up to one month.

HEALTHY NOTE

Using low-fat mayonnaise makes the fat content of this hummus lower than with the traditional recipe.

Olive Tapenade with Lemon

Use olive tapenade as a relish to add zest and a Mediterranean flavor to many foods.

Yield:	Prep time:	Cook time:	Serving size:
1¼ cups	10 minutes	None	2 tablespoons

Each serving has:				
69 calories	7 g total fat	1 g saturated fat	1 mg cholesterol	228 mg sodium
1.5 g carbohydrates	0.6 g fiber	0 g sugars	0.7 g protein	

1 cup pitted kalamata olives	1 TB. lemon zest, finely grated
1½ tsp. garlic, minced	2 TB. lemon juice
4 anchovy fillets	¼ cup extra-virgin olive oil
2 TB. capers	2 TB. fresh parsley, chopped

1. Place olives, garlic, anchovies, capers, lemon zest, and lemon juice in a food processor. Process until mixture is blended. With the processor running, slowly pour in oil.

2. Transfer to a medium bowl and fold in parsley. Refrigerate in an airtight container for up to 10 days.

TABLE TALK

Use this tangy condiment as a spread for flax seed crackers or vegetable scoopers. You can also use it to top fish, eggs, ham, or chicken. It's zesty and intense, so a little can add plenty of interest to your meal.

Curry Cashew Dip

Use this dip with grilled meats and vegetables and with vegetable scoopers. Ginger and chutney enhance the curry flavor.

Yield:	Prep time:	Cook time:	Serving size:
⅔ cup	10 minutes	None	2 tablespoons

Each serving has:				
121 calories	9.2 g total fat	1.7 g saturated fat	0 mg cholesterol	186 mg sodium
8.2 g carbohydrates	0.7 g fiber	3.1 g sugars	2.3 g protein	

½ cup raw, unsalted cashews	1 shallot, chopped
1 TB. olive oil	1 tsp. curry powder
1 TB. chutney or all-natural fruit preserves	¼ tsp. salt
	⅛ tsp. chili powder
1 TB. rice vinegar	2 TB. water
1 TB. fresh ginger, chopped	

1. Place cashews, oil, chutney or preserves, vinegar, ginger, shallot, curry powder, salt, chili pepper, and water in a food processor. Process until thick but not smooth. Serve at once or store in an airtight container in the refrigerator for up to 3 months.

TABLE TALK

Cashews make a tasty nut butter all by themselves. Process ¾ cup roasted cashews until they turn into butter in a food processor. Serve as you would any nut butter.

Salmon Mousse

Serve this elegant, high-omega-3 mousse as an appetizer, a late-afternoon snack, or a light lunch. The flavors of horseradish and dill will give you much taste satisfaction.

Yield:	Prep time:	Cook time:	Serving size:
4 cups	15 minutes plus 3 hours chill time	None	½ cup

Each serving has:				
149 calories	7.1 g total fat	1.8 g saturated fat	36 mg cholesterol	227 mg sodium
4.6 g carbohydrates	0 g fiber	3.7 g sugars	15.2 g protein	

1 envelope unflavored gelatin	1 TB. lemon juice
½ cup hot water	½ tsp. salt
1½ cups plain low-fat yogurt	1 can (14.75-oz.) pink salmon, drained and skin removed
2 TB. prepared horseradish	
2 TB. green onion, finely chopped	2 TB. chives, snipped
2½ tsp. lemon zest, grated	2 TB. dill, snipped

1. Place gelatin in a heatproof glass measuring cup or bowl. Add hot water and stir until dissolved.

2. In a food processor, blend yogurt, horseradish, onion, lemon zest, lemon juice, and salt. Remove and place in a medium bowl.

3. With a fork, gently flake salmon into small pieces. Stir salmon and gelatin into yogurt mixture.

4. Transfer to a 4-cup bowl or decorative mold, cover, and refrigerate 3 hours or more for mousse to set. Unmold onto a platter to serve. Garnish with chives and dill.

HEALTHY NOTE

Salmon is a cold-water fish that's very high in important omega-3 essential fatty acids. This mousse is low in fat and high in inflammation-lowering ingredients.

Baked Yam Skins

Yam skins are the healthful alternative to baked white potato skins. These are crunchy, spicy, and cheese filled.

Yield:	Prep time:	Cook time:	Serving size:
12 wedges	10 minutes	1 hour 25 minutes	2 skins

Each serving has:				
82 calories	3 g total fat	0.7 g saturated fat	2 mg cholesterol	63 mg sodium
10.8 g carbohydrates	1.6 g fiber	0 g sugars	2.9 g protein	

3 yams (8 oz. each), washed and dried	½ cup (2-oz.) low-fat Monterrey Jack cheese
1 TB. olive oil	½ tsp. chili powder

1. Preheat the oven to 425°F.

2. Place yams on a foil-lined baking sheet and bake for 1 hour or until fork-tender but not mushy. Reduce the oven temperature to 400°F.

3. When yams are cool enough to handle, halve lengthwise and scoop out most of the flesh, leaving a ¼-inch shell. Then halve yam skins lengthwise again so you have 12 skins total.

4. Drizzle olive oil over flesh side of yam skins. Bake, flesh side down, for 20 minutes.

5. Turn yam skins flesh side up and sprinkle with cheese and chili powder. Bake for 5 more minutes or until skins are crisp and cheese has melted. You can bake the yams a day or two early and store in the refrigerator until you're ready to bake the skins.

TABLE TALK

Use the leftover flesh of these yams for mashed yams. Make them savory by adding a teaspoon of garlic and a tablespoon of olive oil and topping with a sprinkle of Parmesan cheese. Or serve them with the sweet flavors of a tablespoon of olive oil and a dash of cinnamon.

Figs with Ricotta Spread

Tender figs blend with ricotta, basil, and walnuts to give you a sweet spread to serve on cucumber slices.

Yield:	Prep time:	Cook time:	Serving size:
1½ cups	15 minutes	None	2 tablespoons

Each serving has:				
90 calories	3.8 g total fat	0 g saturated fat	4 mg cholesterol	25 mg sodium
11.7 g carbohydrates	2.1 g fiber	8.2 g sugars	4.2 g protein	

¾ cup dried figs, cut in quarters

2 cups boiling water

¾ cup low-fat ricotta, crumbled

½ cup no-fat sour cream

3 TB. fresh basil, snipped

2 TB. water

½ cup walnuts, toasted and chopped

2 cucumbers, sliced

1. In a small bowl, pour boiling water over figs. Let stand for 15 minutes and then drain.

2. While figs are soaking, in a medium bowl, stir together ricotta, sour cream, basil, and water. Stir in drained figs and ¼ cup walnuts. Spread may be chilled at this point for up to 24 hours.

3. To serve, transfer spread to a serving bowl. Top with remaining ¼ cup walnuts. Serve with cucumbers.

HEALTHY NOTE

The sugar nutritional count in this recipe comes exclusively from the figs. Figs offer dietary fiber, potassium, and manganese. This sugar isn't empty calories, but rather a natural sugar that provides excellent nutritional value.

Spicy Coriander Pecans

Let these pecans transport your taste buds to the exotic Middle East as you savor the spices of cumin, coriander, cayenne, and ginger.

Yield:	Prep time:	Cook time:	Serving size:
4 cups	10 minutes	25-40 minutes	¼ cup

Each serving has:				
193 calories	19.5 g total fat	1.7 g saturated fat	0 mg cholesterol	78 mg sodium
5.1 g carbohydrates	2.7 g fiber	2.2 g sugars	2.8 g protein	

1 egg white	1½ tsp. ground cumin
1 TB. water	1 tsp. paprika
4 cups raw whole pecan halves	1 tsp. ground coriander
2 TB. brown sugar	½ tsp. cayenne pepper
½ tsp. salt	¼ tsp. ground ginger

1. Preheat oven to 300°F. In a medium bowl, beat egg white and water until frothy. Add pecans and toss to coat. Transfer to a wire-mesh sieve; drain pecans for 5 minutes.

2. While the nuts drain, in a large plastic bag, combine brown sugar, salt, cumin, paprika, coriander, cayenne pepper, and ginger. Add nuts to bag and shake well to coat. Spread nuts evenly in an ungreased 15×10×1-inch baking pan.

3. Bake for 35 to 40 minutes until nuts are toasted and spice mixture is dry, stirring every 10 minutes. Remove from oven and transfer to a sheet of foil. Cool completely. Break apart. Store in airtight bag or container at room temperature up to 5 days, or freeze up to 3 months.

Variation: Substitute walnuts or almonds for pecans.

HEALTHY NOTE

Pecans are high in oleic oils, fiber, and vitamin E.

Smoked Trout Spread

You'll enjoy this spread for the taste, while your health will enjoy it for the high amounts of minerals and vitamins in every bite.

Yield:	Prep time:	Cook time:	Serving size:
1¾ cups	10 minutes	None	2 tablespoons

Each serving has:				
55 calories	1.7 g total fat	0 g saturated fat	13 mg cholesterol	82 mg sodium
3.1 g carbohydrates	0.6 g fiber	1.6 g sugars	6.6 g protein	

2 (3-oz.) pkg. low-fat cream cheese, softened

¼ cup low-fat plain yogurt

3 TB. green onion, finely chopped

1½ tsp. lemon zest, finely shredded

3 TB. lemon juice

¼ tsp. freshly ground black pepper

8 oz. smoked trout fillets (or other smoked whitefish), skin and bones removed and flaked

Fresh chives or chopped green onion (optional)

3 medium red bell peppers, seeded, cored, and cut into 1-in.-wide strips

1. In a medium bowl, stir together cream cheese, yogurt, onion, lemon zest, lemon juice, and black pepper until well combined. Gently fold in trout.

2. Transfer spread to a small serving bowl. Top with chives or onion, if using. Serve with bell pepper strips. Can be covered and refrigerated for up to 3 days.

Variation: Substitute smoked salmon or chipped beef for the trout.

TABLE TALK

Try this excellent healthy snack for a late-afternoon pick-me-up, as a special treat for your child's lunchbox, or as a game-day appetizer.

Nut Butter

Whether you make yours creamy or chunky, the delicious flavor of nut butters will enliven your snacks.

Yield:	Prep time:	Cook time:	Serving size:
1 cup	6 minutes	None	2 tablespoons

Each serving has:				
51 calories	4.4 g total fat	0 g saturated fat	13 mg cholesterol	82 mg sodium
0.8 g carbohydrates	1.1 g fiber	0 g sugars	1.9 g protein	

¾ cup nuts, either cashews,
     almonds, macadamias,
     hazelnuts, or peanuts

1. Place nuts in a food processor and process in bursts until nuts form a chunky or creamy butter, about 2 to 4 minutes.

2. Store in an airtight container in the refrigerator for up to 6 months.

TABLE TALK

Walnuts or pecans can be processed into nut butters but be prepared—they are astringent and don't have a sweet taste as other nuts do.

Soups and Stews

In This Chapter

- Soothing body and spirit with soups
- Making hot meaty stews and chilled summer soups
- Using the healthiest ingredients
- Adding anti-inflammatory spices and herbs

Preparing and eating soups gives you a fabulous opportunity to experiment with many anti-inflammatory ingredients. The success of your soups depends on using the freshest organic ingredients and the leanest drug-free meats, poultry, and fish.

The *piece de resistance* of a delicious soup is the seasoning, which brings a complementary flavor to your mouth that's irresistible.

Some of the spices and herbs you'll find in these recipes include rosemary, garlic, parsley, thyme, cayenne, cilantro, chives, basil, oregano, lemongrass, and ginger. If you can, grow these in your garden or on a window sill and harvest them fresh. The intensity of the taste and the fragrance will delight your culinary senses. If you don't grow them, purchase them fresh. Otherwise, go ahead and use the dried versions—they'll still add enticing flavor.

Other herbs and spices include chipotle chili, freshly ground black pepper, celery seed, horseradish, bay leaves, and capers. Black pepper tastes best when freshly ground. Be sure to remove bay leaves before serving the soup—they're for flavoring only, not for eating. Capers are a pickled form of fresh black pepper.

If we haven't included your favorite seasoning in these recipes, go ahead—be daring and add it anyway. It will enhance your cooking and eating experience.

Artichoke and Chicken Soup

Garlic and lemon juice add flavor to artichoke and chicken soup.

Yield:	Prep time:	Cook time:	Serving size:
8 cups	15 minutes	35 minutes	2 cups

Each serving has:				
320 calories	9.8 g total fat	2.3 g saturated fat	6 mg cholesterol	292 mg sodium
51.1 g carbohydrates	12.3 g fiber	3 g sugars	11.8 g protein	

4¼ cups water

¾ cup brown rice

2 TB. olive oil

1 tsp. garlic, minced

2 (14-oz.) cans artichoke hearts, drained and quartered

3 TB. lemon juice

1 white or yellow small onion, chopped

¼ cup Parmesan cheese, grated

1. Bring 2 cups water to a boil in a medium saucepan. Add rice, cover, and cook at a gentle boil while preparing other ingredients.

2. Heat oil in a large skillet over medium-high heat. Add garlic and artichoke, and sauté for 5 to 6 minutes. Add lemon juice and set aside.

3. In the same skillet, add onions and sauté for 2 to 3 minutes.

4. When rice is cooked, add remaining 2¼ cups water, artichoke mixture, and onions to the saucepan. Heat to boiling. Transfer to a serving dish and top with Parmesan cheese. Serve hot.

HEALTHY NOTE

Preparing this high-fiber soup with water and not chicken broth significantly reduces your sodium intake yet offers delicious eating.

Fish Stew with Vegetables

Vegetables add a healthy glow to the fish stew flavored with lemon and garlic.

Yield:	Prep time:	Cook time:	Serving size:
10 cups	20 minutes	30 minutes	1²/₃ cups

Each serving has:				
258 calories	7.8 g total fat	1.6 g saturated fat	65 mg cholesterol	370 mg sodium
4 g carbohydrates	10 g fiber	2 g sugars	41 g protein	

6 cups water	1 TB. olive oil
2 lb. fish (such as halibut, prawns, salmon, tuna, or clams)	1 medium white or yellow onion, chopped
¹/₂ lemon, sliced	1 tsp. garlic, minced
1 stalk celery, coarsely chopped	¹/₄ cup tomato sauce
1 carrot, coarsely chopped	¹/₂ tsp. salt
1 medium tomato, coarsely chopped	¹/₄ tsp. freshly ground black pepper
¹/₂ TB. butter	3 TB. parsley, chopped

1. Bring water to a boil in a medium saucepan over high heat. Add fish, lemon, celery, carrot, and tomato to pan, and cook for 5 minutes.

2. Drain fish, retaining fish stock and vegetables. Heat butter and oil in a large skillet over medium heat.

3. Add onion and garlic to skillet and sauté for 2 minutes. Add tomato sauce and cook for another 10 minutes. Add salt and pepper.

4. Place the fish, garlic, onion, tomatoes, and vegetables in the skillet. Cook for another 5 minutes.

5. Sprinkle with parsley and serve.

TABLE TALK

The fat content of the recipe changes based on the type of fish you choose. The nutritional counts for this recipe were calculated using halibut.

Pumpkin Soup

This savory soup is a delicious and different way to eat healthy pumpkin.

Yield:	Prep time:	Cook time:	Serving size:
8 cups	15 minutes	2 to 10 minutes	$1\frac{1}{3}$ cups

Each serving has:				
78 calories	3.6 g total fat	2 g saturated fat	7 mg cholesterol	441 mg sodium
7.9 g carbohydrates	2.7 g fiber	3.1 g sugars	4.5 g protein	

1 TB. butter

1 stalk celery, chopped

1 tsp. garlic, minced

2 cups prepared pumpkin purée or
    canned pumpkin

3 cups vegetable broth

3 cups water

$\frac{1}{4}$ tsp. freshly ground black pepper

2 TB. fresh parsley, chopped

2 TB. fresh basil, chopped

1 TB. fresh thyme, chopped

3 TB. Parmesan cheese, grated

1. In a large saucepan, melt butter. Add celery and garlic, and sauté approximately 2 to 3 minutes over medium heat. Slowly stir in pumpkin, vegetable broth, water, and pepper.

2. Bring soup to a boil, and then simmer for 2 to 10 minutes until hot throughout. Stir in parsley, basil, and thyme. Ladle into 6 serving bowls and top each with $\frac{1}{2}$ tablespoon grated Parmesan cheese. Serve hot.

HEALTHY NOTE

Pumpkin's bright orange color indicates that it is high in beta-carotene. This important antioxidant may reduce the risk of developing certain types of cancer and offers protection against heart disease. It also gives skin a healthy glow.

Veal Stew with Yams

Veal and yams blend flavors to make this tomato-based entrée.

Yield:	Prep time:	Cook time:	Serving size:
1½ pounds veal and 4½ cups vegetables	20 minutes	45 minutes	4 ounces veal and ¾ cup vegetables

Each serving has:				
278 g calories	6.2 mg total fat	1.8 mg saturated fat	125 g cholesterol	224 g sodium
19.7 g carbohydrates	3.1 g fiber	2.7 g sugars	31.9 g protein	

½ TB. butter

1 TB. olive oil

1 carrot, thinly sliced

1 medium yellow onion, thinly sliced

1½ lb. lean veal, all visible fat removed and diced

½ cup white wine

⅓ cup tomato sauce

¼ tsp. salt

⅛ tsp. pepper

4 medium yams, cut in quarters

2 cups water or enough to cover veal and yams

1. In a large skillet, heat butter and olive oil. Add carrot and onion, and sauté 2 to 3 minutes. Add veal and cook until lightly browned.

2. Remove veal to a side platter. Add white wine, tomato sauce, salt, and pepper to skillet.

3. When liquid has reduced by about half, add yams to the skillet. Cover with water and cook uncovered for 30 minutes. Add veal and cook for an additional 15 minutes.

4. When meat and yams are tender, the dish is ready. Serve immediately.

TABLE TALK

If veal is unavailable, you can make this stew with trimmed beef. Substitute water and one teaspoon balsamic vinegar for the white wine, if you prefer.

Mediterranean Shrimp Stew

Oregano and capers add zest to shrimp, tomatoes, and carrots.

Yield:	Prep time:	Cook time:	Serving size:
8 cups	15 minutes	15 minutes	1⅓ cups

Each serving has:				
165 calories	3.3 g total fat	3.3 g saturated fat	223 mg cholesterol	402 mg sodium
8.4 g carbohydrates	2.7 g fiber	4.1 g sugars	26.5 g protein	

2 tsp. olive oil	3 medium tomatoes, chopped
1 tsp. garlic, minced	2 TB. capers, drained
3 medium carrots, chopped	3 cups low-sodium vegetable broth
2 small red or yellow potatoes, unpeeled and chopped	1½ lb. medium shrimp, peeled and deveined
2 TB. fresh oregano, chopped	¼ tsp. freshly ground black pepper

1. In a 4-quart pot, heat oil over medium heat. Add garlic, carrots, potatoes, and oregano. Sauté for 2 minutes. Add tomatoes, capers, and broth. Increase heat to high, to bring mixture to a boil. Reduce heat to medium-low, cover, and cook for 10 minutes or more until potatoes are soft.

2. Mash several potato chunks with a fork to thicken soup, leaving most of the pieces intact. Add shrimp, stir, and cover for 2 minutes, cooking until shrimp are pink and cooked through. Stir in pepper and serve warm.

Variation: Substitute salmon or clams for shrimp.

TABLE TALK

Oregano is used as a flavoring in many classic Mediterranean dishes. Crush it by hand to release its full flavor and aroma. You can grow oregano easily in an herb garden outdoors or on a window sill.

Moroccan Beef Stew

Vegetables add balance to this beef stew that's flavored with cayenne, garlic, and bay leaves.

Yield:	Prep time:	Cook time:	Serving size:
9 cups	40 minutes	2 hours	1½ cups

Each serving has:				
297 calories	11 g total fat	3.3 g saturated fat	79 mg cholesterol	260 mg sodium
13.9 g carbohydrates	3.9 g fiber	5 g sugars	33.5 g protein	

1¼ lb. top round roast, trimmed and cut into 1-in. cubes

1 tsp. smoked paprika

¼ tsp. salt

¼ tsp. cayenne pepper

1 TB. olive oil

1 medium white onion, chopped

¼ tsp. dried thyme

¼ tsp. dried oregano

2 TB. low-sodium tomato paste

3 tsp. garlic, minced

2 TB. whole-wheat flour

4 TB. balsamic vinegar

2½ cups low-sodium vegetable broth

2 bay leaves

3 carrots, cut into ½-in. pieces

2 cups celery, coarsely chopped

1 cup frozen peas

1. Pat beef dry with a paper towel and sprinkle with paprika, salt, and cayenne pepper. In a large, heavy pot or Dutch oven, heat ½ tablespoon oil on medium-high heat. Add half of beef and cook until browned. Transfer to a large plate. Repeat with remaining ½ tablespoon oil and beef, and transfer to the same large plate.

2. Add onion to the pot and sauté until soft and lightly browned, about 6 minutes. Reduce heat to medium-low and stir in thyme, oregano, tomato paste, and garlic.

3. Return beef and any juices to the pot. Sprinkle with flour and cook for 1 minute, stirring constantly. Add vinegar, broth, and bay leaves. Cover and increase heat to medium-high. Bring to slow simmer and cook for 1 hour and 15 minutes, stirring 2 to 3 times.

4. Add carrots and simmer for 30 minutes. Add celery, cover, and simmer until vegetables and beef are tender, 10 to 20 minutes.

5. Add peas and cook until just heated through, 1 to 2 minutes. Remove bay leaves and serve immediately.

Gazpacho with Pecans

This cool summer treat sizzles with a tangy base of red wine vinegar and garlic.

Yield:	Prep time:	Cook time:	Serving size:
6 cups	10 minutes plus 2 hours chill time	None	1 cup

Each serving has:				
179 calories	16.7 g total fat	1.8 g saturated fat	1.8 mg cholesterol	11 mg sodium
7.5 g carbohydrates	2.5 g fiber	3.2 g sugars	2.3 g protein	

2 small tomatoes, seeded and finely chopped	3 TB. olive oil
2 stalks celery, finely chopped	¼ cup red wine vinegar
1 cucumber, finely chopped	1 clove garlic, minced
1 medium red onion, finely chopped	2 tsp. lemon zest, finely grated
½ cup fresh flat-leaf parsley, coarsely chopped	¾ cup toasted pecans, coarsely chopped

1. Combine tomatoes, celery, cucumber, onion, and parsley in a medium bowl. Whisk oil, vinegar, garlic, and lemon zest in a small bowl until dressing is combined. Stir dressing into vegetable mixture.

2. Cover the bowl and refrigerate for at least 2 hours. Stir in nuts before serving.

TABLE TALK

If you like the taste and texture of wet nuts, add the pecans to the gazpacho before chilling. You can also substitute walnuts to add omega-3 fatty acids to the soup.

Chicken Avocado Soup

This is a light and tasty soup with Southwestern flavors that you can serve with virtually any entrée and grilled meats.

Yield:	Prep time:	Cook time:	Serving size:
8 cups	5 minutes	15 minutes	1⅓ cups

Each serving has:				
168 calories	6.9 g total fat	1.3 g saturated fat	48 mg cholesterol	119 mg sodium
5.2 g carbohydrates	2.5 g fiber	0 g sugars	20.6 g protein	

6¼ cups low-sodium chicken stock

2 tsp. garlic, finely chopped

1 dried chipotle chili, cut into thin strips

1 avocado

2 TB. lime juice

3 green onions, thinly sliced

12 oz. cooked chicken breast meat, cut into shreds or thin strips

2 TB. fresh cilantro, chopped

1 lime, cut into wedges

1. Place stock in a large, heavy-bottom pan with garlic and chili strips and bring to a boil over high heat.

2. Meanwhile, cut avocado in half around the pit. Twist apart and then remove the pit with a knife. Carefully peel off skin, dice flesh, and place in a small bowl. Sprinkle with lime juice and toss to prevent discoloration (oxidation).

3. Arrange green onions, chicken, avocado, and cilantro in the bottom of 6 soup bowls. Ladle hot stock into the bowls and serve with lime wedges.

HEALTHY NOTE

The avocado is a super anti-inflammatory fruit. While being high in fat, it's also high in fiber and monounsaturated fats.

Thai Shrimp Coconut Soup

You'll be delighted with the authentic Thai flavor and taste of this coconut-based soup.

Yield:	Prep time:	Cook time:	Serving size:
10 cups	10 minutes	20 minutes	1⅔ cups

Each serving has:				
246 calories	10.5 g total fat	8.7 g saturated fat	147 mg cholesterol	457 mg sodium
20.6 g carbohydrates	1.6 g fiber	2.2 g sugars	18 g protein	

4 oz. dried cellophane noodles	1 lb. fresh shrimp, deveined
5 cups low-sodium chicken or vegetable stock	1 cup unsweetened coconut milk
1 lemongrass stalk, crushed	2 TB. nam pla (Thai fish sauce)
½-in. piece fresh gingerroot, peeled and finely chopped	1 TB. lime juice
1 fresh red chili, seeded and thinly sliced	½ cup bean sprouts
	4 TB. green onions, finely sliced
	Fresh cilantro leaves

1. Soak noodles in a large bowl, with enough lukewarm water to cover, for 20 minutes until soft, or cook according to the package instructions. Drain well and set aside.

2. Meanwhile, bring stock to a boil in a large pan over high heat. Lower the heat; add lemongrass, gingerroot, and chili; and simmer for 5 minutes. Add shrimp and continue to simmer for an additional 3 minutes or until shrimp is cooked. Remove shrimp to a side plate.

3. Stir in coconut milk, nam pla, and lime juice, and continue simmering for 3 minutes. Add bean sprouts and green onions, and simmer for another 1 minute. Remove and discard lemongrass stalk.

4. Divide noodles among 6 bowls. Bring soup back to a boil and then add soup to each bowl. Divide shrimp equally among the bowls. The heat of the soup will warm the noodles. To garnish, sprinkle with cilantro leaves.

TABLE TALK

Lemongrass lends a delightful Thai character to this soup. It's widely available at most grocery stores.

Chilled Avocado Soup

Healthy yogurt is the base of this creamy and rich-tasting soup.

Yield:	Prep time:	Cook time:	Serving size:
3 cups	10 minutes	None	½ cup

Each serving has:				
190 calories	15.2 g total fat	2.5 g saturated fat	3 mg cholesterol	235 mg sodium
12.6 g carbohydrates	6.8 g fiber	2.8 g sugars	4.4 g protein	

3 ripe avocados	1 (8-oz.) carton low-fat plain yogurt
4 TB. fresh lemon juice	¼ tsp. salt
1 (10-oz.) can reduced-sodium chicken broth	¼ tsp. cayenne
	3 TB. chives, chopped

1. Peel avocados, remove pits, and add to the blender with lemon juice, chicken broth, and yogurt. Process until smooth.

2. Add salt and cayenne, and refrigerate for several hours. Serve in soup bowls with chives on top.

TABLE TALK

Serve this creamy, rich soup with a fresh main-dish salad or with grilled or broiled fish or meat.

Carrot Tomato Soup

Apricots lend sweetness to this puréed vegetable soup.

Yield:	Prep time:	Cook time:	Serving size:
6 cups	20 minutes	10 minutes	1 cup

Each serving has:				
63 calories	1.8 g total fat	1 g saturated fat	5 mg cholesterol	64 mg sodium
11.4 g carbohydrates	2.5 g fiber	6.1 g sugars	1.6 g protein	

$\frac{1}{3}$ cup dried apricots, finely chopped	1 cup low-sodium tomato juice
1 cup boiling water	$\frac{1}{2}$ cup water
1 (16-oz.) package shredded carrots	$\frac{1}{4}$ cup lemon juice
	$\frac{1}{3}$ cup low-fat sour cream

1. Soak apricots in boiling water for 15 minutes, to soften.

2. Combine carrots, tomato juice, apricots with soaking water, and $\frac{1}{2}$ cup water in a large casserole dish. Microwave on high for 10 minutes until mixture boils; then remove and let sit for 5 minutes.

3. Using a blender or food processor, process mixture until smooth. Return to the casserole dish.

4. Add lemon juice and sour cream, and stir well. Serve at room temperature or chilled.

TABLE TALK

If you prefer a soup with more texture, omit using the food processor.

Barley Soup with Vegetables

Barley hosts a plethora of healthy vegetables with flavorings of bay leaf, thyme, and garlic.

Yield:	Prep time:	Cook time:	Serving size:
16 cups	20 minutes	55 minutes	2 cups

Each serving has:				
164 calories	5.6 g total fat	0.8 g saturated fat	0 mg cholesterol	245 mg sodium
24.2 g carbohydrates	5.8 g fiber	6 g sugars	5.5 g protein	

3 TB. olive oil

2 medium yellow onions, coarsely chopped

2 tsp. garlic, minced

4 carrots, sliced in $\frac{1}{2}$-in. pieces

3 celery stalks with leaves, chopped in $\frac{1}{2}$-in. pieces

1 large yam, chopped in $\frac{3}{4}$-in. cubes

2 small zucchini, chopped in $\frac{1}{2}$-in. pieces

2 cups green beans, chopped in 1-in. pieces

7 cups low-sodium chicken broth

2 medium tomatoes, coarsely chopped

1 bay leaf

$\frac{1}{2}$ tsp. salt

$\frac{1}{4}$ tsp. pepper

$\frac{3}{4}$ cup fresh spinach leaves, finely shredded

1 cup cooked barley

1 tsp. dried thyme

1. In a large soup pot, heat oil over medium-high heat. Add onions and garlic, and cook until translucent, about 5 minutes.

2. Add carrots, celery, yam, zucchini, and beans. Stir in broth and tomatoes, and bring to a boil. Reduce heat and add bay leaf, salt, and pepper. Cover and simmer for 45 minutes.

3. Discard bay leaf. Stir in spinach, barley, and thyme.

4. Adjust seasonings, if desired. Simmer for 5 minutes or until heated through.

TABLE TALK

This soup is wonderful as a vegetarian meal served with cheese and crackers or with one of the appetizer or snacks in Chapter 7.

Jicama and Corn Gazpacho

Jicama and cucumber add crunch to this tomato-based cold soup.

Yield:	Prep time:	Cook time:	Serving size:
6 cups	25 minutes plus 1 hour chill time	None	1 cup

Each serving has:

78 calories	0.8 g total fat	0 g saturated fat	0 mg cholesterol	138 mg sodium
17.5 g carbohydrates	4.8 g fiber	5.8 g sugars	2.7 g protein	

2 large tomatoes, quartered and seeded	2 cups jicama, peeled and chopped
1 cup carrot juice	$\frac{1}{2}$ cup arugula, shredded
$\frac{1}{2}$ cup water	2 TB. prepared horseradish
2 TB. fresh chives, coarsely chopped	$\frac{1}{2}$ tsp. salt
1 medium cucumber, seeded and coarsely chopped	4 large or 6 small radishes, quartered
$1\frac{1}{2}$ cups fresh or frozen corn kernels	2 limes, cut into wedges

1. In a blender or food processor, combine tomatoes, carrot juice, water, and chives. Blend or process until smooth.

2. Transfer mixture to a large bowl. Stir in cucumber, corn, jicama, arugula, horseradish, and salt. Cover and refrigerate at least 1 hour or up to 24 hours before serving.

3. Ladle soup into bowls or glasses. Top with radishes and serve with lime wedges.

TABLE TALK

Jicama is a large root bulb that is crisp and fresh tasting. It adds a juicy crunch to this gazpacho.

Richly Tomato Soup

Not your everyday tomato soup, this one contains three sources of tomatoes flavored with Italian parsley and celery seed.

Yield:	Prep time:	Cook time:	Serving size:
6 cups	15 minutes	35 minutes	1 cup

Each serving has:				
86 calories	3.1 g total fat	0.5 g saturated fat	0 mg cholesterol	279 mg sodium
11.8 g carbohydrates	3.4 g fiber	7.2 g sugars	3.8 g protein	

1 TB. olive oil

1 large white onion, sliced

1 (28-oz.) can whole tomatoes, undrained

¾ cup dried tomatoes (not oil packed), divided

½ (6-oz.) can no-salt-added tomato paste

1½ cups reduced-sodium vegetable broth

½ cup (1 stalk) sliced celery

½ tsp. celery seed

4 TB. fresh Italian (flat-leaf) parsley, snipped

1 TB. lemon juice

1. Heat oil in a 4-quart Dutch oven. Cook onion in hot oil, covered, over medium-low heat for 10 minutes or until tender.

2. Add undrained tomatoes, ½ cup dried tomatoes, tomato paste, broth, celery, celery seed, and 2 tablespoons parsley. Bring to a boil. Reduce heat. Simmer, covered, for 20 minutes. Set aside to cool.

3. Meanwhile, place ¼ cup dried tomatoes in a microwave-safe bowl and cover with water. Cook on high for 1 minute. Cool. Drain and snip into pieces. Set aside.

4. In a food processor, process half the broth–tomato mixture at a time until smooth. Return to saucepan. Add lemon juice and heat to serving temperature.

5. Ladle soup into 6 bowls and top with snipped dried tomatoes and remaining 2 tablespoons parsley.

TABLE TALK

Using three different types of tomato products intensifies the tomato taste of this soup.

Main Course Entrées

The dinner meal needs to offer you appealing foods that fight inflammation. Our recipes do just that. You'll be cooking with the highest-quality meats, poultry, and seafood. One of the biggest inflammation-fighting features of these recipes is the spices, herbs, and seasonings that do double duty. They give you sparkling and savory mouthwatering flavor, while their special antioxidant and soothing components calm your body.

Our many seafood offerings focus on fish and shellfish that give your omega-3 essential fatty acid intake a healthy boost. You'll be preparing meals in traditional American and varied ethnic cuisines.

You'll find intriguing and appealing vegetarian main dishes that work whether you're a committed vegetarian or you simply enjoy a nonmeat meal several times a week.

Beef and Pork Main Dishes

In This Chapter

- Preparing meat in anti-inflammatory ways
- Eating drug-free, healthful meats
- Lowering the saturated fat content of meals that include meat
- Benefiting from the high concentrations of minerals and B-vitamins in healthful meats

Eating meat on an anti-inflammatory diet can be challenging. You want to maximize the nutritional benefits of meat, which include these:

- High amounts of complete and easily digested protein
- High concentration of minerals and B-vitamins
- High amounts of CLA (conjugated linoleic acid)
- Terrific robust tastes

At the same time, you want to minimize the possible disadvantages of saturated fat, cholesterol, and additives such as growth hormones.

Our recipes achieve these goals by giving you some helpful directions:

- Use drug-free, grass-fed, organic meats
- Trim away all visible fat
- Use only lean cuts of meat
- Cook meats in ways that reduce fat content

Enjoy!

Italian Pork Loin with Mushrooms

Lean tenderloin is rubbed with rosemary, garlic, sage, and fennel seeds, and then grilled until tender. It's served with vegetables in a flavorful balsamic vinaigrette reduction sauce.

Yield:	Prep time:	Cook time:	Serving size:
1 pork loin and 4 cups vegetables	30 minutes, plus overnight	12 to 15 minutes	0.3 pound pork and ²/₃ cup vegetables

Each serving has:				
239 calories	7.3 g total fat	2 g saturated fat	97 mg cholesterol	331 mg sodium
4.5 g carbohydrates	1.3 g fiber	1.9 g sugars	36.6 g protein	

1 tsp. dried rosemary	6 oz. crimini mushrooms
2 tsp. garlic, minced	1 cup carrot, cut into ½-in. slices
1 tsp. dried sage	1 cup celery, cut into ½-in. slices
1 tsp. fennel seeds	1 tsp. fresh parsley, chopped
¼ tsp. salt	1 TB. olive oil
¼ tsp. freshly ground black pepper	3 TB. balsamic vinegar
1¾ lb. pork tenderloin	1 cup vegetable broth

1. Chop rosemary, garlic, sage, and fennel seeds together; add salt and black pepper to the mixture.

2. Make small shallow holes about 1 inch apart in pork tenderloin with a fine-blade knife. Insert spice mixture into the holes. Place pork in a zipper-lock plastic bag and place in the refrigerator overnight.

3. The next day, heat the grill to medium-high and grill pork tenderloin for 12 to 15 minutes, turning once. Cook pork to 160°F on a meat thermometer.

4. While pork is grilling, in a large skillet, sauté mushrooms, carrots, celery, and parsley in olive oil for 5 to 10 minutes, until al dente. Add vinegar and vegetable broth, and cook until it reduces, 10 to 15 minutes.

5. Slice grilled pork and arrange on a serving plate along with cooked vegetables.

TABLE TALK

The rub for the pork tenderloin contains traditional Italian spices that makes this dish authentic. You could also use this rub for seasoning pasta or topping garlic bread.

Beef Filet with Balsamic Vinegar

This simple-to-make recipe will delight your taste buds with its tangy-sweet sauce. Add a crisp romaine salad as a side dish.

Yield:	Prep time:	Cook time:	Serving size:
1¾ pounds beef	5 minutes	10 to 20 minutes	0.3 pound beef

Each serving has:				
275 calories	11.2 g total fat	3.6 g saturated fat	118 mg cholesterol	88 mg sodium
0.1 g carbohydrates	0 g fiber	0 g sugars	40.2 g protein	

1¾ lb. filet of beef, at room temperature	2 TB. plus 1 tsp. olive oil
	¼ cup balsamic vinegar

1. Cut filet into four 1½-inch-thick slices, depending on width of meat. Dry meat with a paper towel.

2. Heat 2 tablespoons oil in a skillet over medium-high and, when it is hot, add filets. Cook on the first side until the bottom is browned to your preferred taste. Flip steaks and cook until juices well up on tops of steaks. This means steak is medium. Remove steaks to a serving platter and let them sit while you deglaze the pan.

3. Remove any fat from the pan, but keep crusty brown bits. Add 1 teaspoon oil. Scrape browned bits into oil with a fork. Add vinegar and cook, stirring, until reduced, about 15 minutes.

4. Pour vinegar reduction on steaks and serve.

TABLE TALK

Balsamic vinegar is slightly sweet, so it adds a tangy yet sweet taste to the meat. You can substitute white or red wine vinegar for a delicious variation.

Beef Goulash

Paprika flavors this authentic goulash, minus the high fat content.

Yield:	Prep time:	Cook time:	Serving size:
1¾ pounds beef	15 minutes	2 ¼ hours	0.3 pound beef

Each serving has:				
311 calories	10.6 g total fat	3.5 g saturated fat	118 mg cholesterol	96 mg sodium
8.6 g carbohydrates	1.3 g fiber	3 g sugars	41.4 g protein	

2 TB. olive oil	¼ cup red wine
1¾ lb. chuck beef, cubed	1 tsp. lemon zest
3 large yellow onions, chopped	1 tsp. dried rosemary
1 tsp. garlic, minced	1 bay leaf
2 TB. all-purpose flour	1 tsp. dried marjoram
2 tsp. paprika	1 oz. tomato paste
1 cup plus 3 TB. water	

1. Place oil, beef, onions, and garlic in a large skillet over medium heat. Sauté to brown meat and soften onions, 5 to 10 minutes.

2. In a small glass, stir together flour and paprika with 3 tablespoons water and pour over meat. Stir to coat meat.

3. Add red wine to the skillet and simmer until it evaporates, and then add lemon zest, rosemary, bay leaf, marjoram, and tomato paste. Stir well. Add 1 cup water, and cover and simmer for at least 2 hours. If goulash becomes too dry, add a little more water.

4. Remove bay leaf and serve at once. You can serve with mixed vegetables, polenta, roasted yams, or mashed cauliflower.

HEALTHY NOTE

Beef gives you great nutritional value: phosphorus, selenium, a plethora of B-vitamins, and zinc. Be sure to trim off any visible fat before cooking, and you can enjoy eating beef a couple times a week. It's healthiest to eat drug-free, grass-fed beef.

Spicy and Sweet Pork

Pomegranate juice flavors this spicy lean pork.

Yield:	Prep time:	Cook time:	Serving size:
1½ pounds pork	10 minutes	23 minutes	¼ pound pork

Each serving has:				
295 calories	13.8 g total fat	3.9 g saturated fat	107 mg cholesterol	269 mg sodium
6.5 g carbohydrates	0 g fiber	5.4 g sugars	33.9 g protein	

½ tsp. ground coriander

½ tsp. ground cinnamon

½ tsp. ground cumin

½ tsp. paprika

½ tsp. salt

2 pork tenderloins (each ¾ lb.), trimmed of visible fat

2 TB. olive oil

1 cup pomegranate juice

2 tsp. balsamic vinegar

1. Preheat oven to 350°F.

2. In a small bowl, stir together coriander, cinnamon, cumin, paprika, and salt. Pat tenderloins dry and rub with spice mixture until evenly distributed.

3. In a large heavy-bottomed skillet, heat oil over medium heat. Add pork and brown on all sides. Transfer pork to a baking dish and place in the oven for about 20 minutes or until a meat thermometer registers 160°F. Remove from the oven and let rest for 10 minutes.

4. Meanwhile, discard any fat from the skillet. Add pomegranate juice to the skillet and boil over medium heat for 2 to 3 minutes or until juice is reduced to about ⅔ cup. Remove from heat and add vinegar.

5. Slice pork on the diagonal and drizzle with pomegranate glaze.

HEALTHY NOTE

Make sure that the pomegranate juice you purchase contains no sugars or artificial sweeteners.

Buffalo Steak and Fries

This buffalo-and-yam-fries combination is flavored with pepper, garlic, and chili powder.

Yield:	Prep time:	Cook time:	Serving size:
1 pound steak and 2 yams	15 minutes	15 to 18 minutes	¼ steak, or 4 ounces, and ½ yam

Each serving has:				
318 calories	4.2 g total fat	0.7 g saturated fat	44 mg cholesterol	76 mg sodium
41.8 g carbohydrates	6.2 g fiber	0.8 g sugars	29.3 g protein	

2 medium yams, cut into french-fry-size strips, about ⅜-in. by ⅜-in., or to your size preference	2 tsp. olive oil
	¼ tsp. salt
1 tsp. garlic powder	¼ tsp. freshly ground black pepper
½ tsp. chili powder	1 lb. buffalo steak

1. Preheat oven to 400°F.

2. Place yams on a baking sheet. Drizzle with 1 teaspoon oil and sprinkle with garlic and chili powders, salt, and pepper, and then toss or mix with your hands to coat. Arrange in a single layer on the baking sheet. Bake fries for 15 to 18 minutes, until lightly browned and crispy.

3. Meanwhile, in a large ovenproof skillet, heat 1 teaspoon oil over medium-high heat. Add steak to skillet and sear on one side, then turn steak over and place the pan in the oven. Cook for 10 to 12 minutes, depending on thickness and desired doneness, until steak is medium-rare to medium.

4. Place steak on a serving plate, arrange fries around steak, and serve immediately.

HEALTHY NOTE

Buffalo is low in fat, cholesterol, and calories compared to beef, yet higher in iron and vitamin B$_{12}$.

Chile Con Carne

Southwestern flavors from cumin, green chilies, and cocoa bring a lively taste to this low-fat chili.

Yield:	Prep time:	Cook time:	Serving size:
8 cups	10 minutes	2 hours	1⅓ cups

Each serving has:				
445 calories	6.6 g total fat	1.5 g saturated fat	34 mg cholesterol	263 mg sodium
67.9 g carbohydrates	18.5 g fiber	16.1 g sugars	31.2 g protein	

1 TB. olive oil	2 tsp. dried oregano
½ lb. beef chuck, trimmed of all visible fat, cut into ½-in. chunks	½ tsp. salt
1 large yellow onion, chopped	1½ tsp. chili powder
2 red bell peppers, cored, seeded, and cut into 1-in. pieces	1 (28-oz.) can diced tomatoes in juice
3 tsp. garlic, minced	1 can green chilies, diced
4 tsp. ground cumin	2 cups water
1 TB. unsweetened cocoa powder	1 (15-oz.) can red kidney beans, rinsed and drained

1. In a large saucepan or Dutch oven, heat oil over medium heat. Add beef and cook until browned, about 5 minutes. With a slotted spoon, transfer beef to a plate.

2. Add onion, bell peppers, and garlic to the pan and cook, stirring frequently, until vegetables are tender, about 15 minutes.

3. Stir in cumin, cocoa powder, oregano, salt, and chili powder, and cook for 1 minute. Add tomatoes in juice, green chilies, beef, and water, and bring to a boil. Reduce to a simmer, cover, and cook for 45 minutes.

4. Stir in beans and cook until beef is tender, 45 minutes to 1 hour.

HEALTHY NOTE

This version of chili con carne delivers great Southwestern taste but with less fat, less cholesterol, and less sodium than the standard recipe.

New Mexican Green Chili

Pork and yams are highlighted with jalapeño pepper, green chilies, and cilantro.

Yield:	Prep time:	Cook time:	Serving size:
9 cups	15 minutes	35 minutes	1½ cups

Each serving has:				
219 calories	7.4 g total fat	1.6 g saturated fat	55 mg cholesterol	131 mg sodium
15.7 g carbohydrates	3.4 g fiber	2.3 g sugars	21.9 g protein	

2 TB. olive oil

1 lb. pork tenderloin, cut into 1-in. chunks

6 green onions, thinly sliced

3 tsp. garlic, minced

1 large green bell pepper, cored, seeded, and cut into ½-in. pieces

1 small jalapeño pepper, finely chopped

2 medium yams, cut into ½-in. chunks

1 (4-oz.) can diced green chilies

1½ cups fresh cilantro, chopped and divided

1¼ cups water

2 TB. lime juice

1. Preheat oven to 350°F. In a large saucepan, heat oil over medium heat. Add pork to the pan and cook until golden brown, about 4 minutes. With a slotted spoon, transfer pork to a plate.

2. Add green onions and garlic to the pan, and cook until onions are tender, about 1 minute. Add bell and jalapeño peppers, and cook about 4 minutes. Stir in yams, chilies, ¾ cup cilantro, and water, and bring to a boil.

3. Return pork to the pan and cover. Place in the oven and bake for 25 minutes or until pork is tender.

4. Stir in lime juice and remaining ¾ cup cilantro. Recover and let stand for 3 minutes before serving.

TABLE TALK

You can turn up the heat in this chili by adding one more jalapeño pepper or by being quite daring and adding a habanero.

Stuffed Burgers

Lean burgers are stuffed with cheddar cheese and flavored with onion and black pepper.

Yield:	Prep time:	Cook time:	Serving size:
6 burgers	10 minutes	10 to 12 minutes	1 burger

Each serving has:				
332 calories	13 g total fat	5.6 g saturated fat	79 mg cholesterol	320 mg sodium
19.6 g carbohydrates	2.9 g fiber	3.6 g sugars	30.9 g protein	

1½ lb. 90% lean ground sirloin or buffalo

½ tsp. freshly ground black pepper

¼ cup white onion, finely chopped

4 oz. low-fat cheddar cheese, shredded

6 whole-wheat hamburger buns

6 iceberg lettuce leaves

6 ¼-in.-thick tomato slices

1. Place ground meat in bowl. Sprinkle with pepper and chopped onions. Divide cheese in 6 equal portions. Form beef around cheese into 6 patties about ¾ inch thick.

2. Grill on medium for 10 minutes. Turn. Grill 10 to 12 minutes more until meat is no longer pink and meat thermometer registers 160°F internal temperature.

3. Toast buns, cut sides down, on grill during last 1 to 2 minutes of grilling. To serve, top bun bottom with lettuce, burger, and tomato. Replace top of bun. Enjoy.

HEALTHY NOTE

These burgers may be somewhat smaller than you normally eat. They contain more than adequate protein for one meal and give you the great taste of beef without overdoing it.

Beef, Barley, and Leeks

This hearty, thyme-flavored stew is perfect for cold weather.

Yield:	Prep time:	Cook time:	Serving size:
8 cups	15 minutes	2 to 5 hours	1⅓ cups

Each serving has:				
321 calories	7.8 g total fat	2.3 g saturated fat	67 mg cholesterol	679 mg sodium
30.8 g carbohydrates	6.7 g fiber	3 g sugars	31 g protein	

1 lb. 90% lean sirloin, cut into 1-in. pieces	3 medium leeks, halved lengthwise and sliced
1 TB. olive oil	2 medium carrots, thinly sliced
1 (49-oz.) can reduced-sodium beef broth	1½ tsp. dried thyme
	¼ tsp. freshly ground black pepper
1 cup regular barley (not quick cooking)	¼ tsp. salt

1. In a large skillet, cook beef in hot oil until browned on all sides. In a 4- to 5-quart slow cooker, combine beef, broth, barley, leeks, carrots, thyme, and pepper.

2. Cover and cook on low heat for 4 to 5 hours or on high heat for 2 to 2½ hours, until barley is tender. Stir in salt. Serve in soup bowls.

TABLE TALK

Beef with barley is a dish featured in pubs throughout Great Britain. It's hearty, tasty, and satisfying.

Mustard Steak with Vegetables

Brown mustard and yogurt sauce is served over sautéed beef, carrots, and onions.

Yield:	Prep time:	Cook time:	Serving size:
2 pounds steak plus 12 cups vegetables	25 minutes	35 minutes	¼ lb. steak and 1½ cups vegetables

Each serving has:				
304 calories	12.2 g total fat	4.3 g saturated fat	82 mg cholesterol	568 mg sodium
16.2 g carbohydrates	3.7 g fiber	3.3 g sugars	31.9 g protein	

½ cup low-fat sour cream

2 TB. coarse-grain brown mustard

1½ lb. boneless beef sirloin steak, trimmed of visible fat

2 TB. olive oil

4 medium carrots, peeled and sliced into ½-in. rounds

1 large red onion, cut into wedges

1 (32-oz.) can reduced-sodium chicken broth

1 lb. yams, cubed

1 lb. fresh spinach

1. Stir together sour cream and mustard; cover and refrigerate.

2. Heat oven to 170°F. Heat a large skillet over medium-high heat. Pat beef dry with paper towels. Heat 1 tablespoon oil in skillet. Add meat and brown in hot skillet for 4 minutes, turning once. Transfer to a platter and set aside.

3. Add remaining 1 tablespoon oil, carrots, and onion to skillet. Cook and stir 5 minutes until browned. Add broth and yams. Bring to a boil and then reduce heat. Cover and cook 15 minutes until tender. Return beef to the skillet. Simmer, covered, for 8 minutes for medium.

4. Reserving broth in a skillet, transfer vegetables and beef to an oven-safe platter. Keep warm in oven. Add spinach to broth and simmer 3 to 4 minutes, tossing with tongs as it cooks.

5. To serve, ladle broth with spinach into 6 small bowls. Divide beef and vegetables among 6 plates. Serve with mustard sauce.

HEALTHY NOTE

This recipe offers you an entire meal with three servings of vegetables.

Ham with Pineapple and Fried Rice

Pineapple adds sweetness to this spicy combination of ham, beans, and rice.

Yield:	Prep time:	Cook time:	Serving size:
6 cups	10 minutes	10 minutes	1 cup

Each serving has:				
360 calories	6.3 g total fat	1.6 g saturated fat	22 g cholesterol	498 mg sodium
59.6 mg carbohydrates	7.8 g fiber	9.3 g sugars	16.7 g protein	

1 TB. olive oil

1 fresh pineapple, peeled, cored, and cut into ¾-in. slices

8 oz. cooked ham, coarsely chopped

1 cup red bell pepper, cored, seeded, and chopped or sliced

1 fresh jalapeño pepper, seeded, if desired, and sliced

½ 15-oz. can black beans, rinsed and drained

1 cup brown rice, cooked

1 lime, cut into wedges

1. Heat oil in a large skillet over medium-high heat. Add pineapple slices and cook 3 to 4 minutes or until beginning to brown. Divide pineapple among four plates.

2. Add ham, bell pepper, and jalapeño to the skillet. Cook 3 minutes, stirring occasionally. Add beans and rice. Cook, stirring occasionally, 3 minutes or until heated through. Divide onto plates with pineapples and serve with lime wedges.

TABLE TALK

This quick stir-fry highlights a Caribbean style of cooking.

Beef Kabobs with Avocado Sauce

Steak cubes are marinated in flavorful oregano and garlic, and served with a mint avocado sauce.

Yield:	Prep time:	Cook time:	Serving size:
8 skewers plus 2 cups avocado sauce	35 minutes	10 to 12 minutes	1 skewer plus ¼ cup avocado sauce

Each serving has:				
297 calories	15.1 g total fat	4.3 g saturated fat	104 mg cholesterol	229 mg sodium
3.5 g carbohydrates	2.1 g fiber	0 g sugars	35.4 g protein	

2 TB. olive oil	½ cup cucumber, coarsely chopped
2 tsp. garlic, minced	⅓ cup fresh mint leaves, lightly packed
1½ tsp. dried oregano, crushed	
1 tsp. freshly ground black pepper	¼ cup low-fat sour cream
2 lb. beef top sirloin steak (about 1 in. thick), trimmed and cut into 1-in. cubes	2 TB. lime juice
	1 TB. water
	½ tsp. salt
1 medium ripe avocado, pitted, peeled, and coarsely chopped	1 tsp. ground cumin

1. In a large bowl, combine oil, garlic, oregano, and pepper. Add meat to oil mixture and toss to coat evenly. Let stand at room temperature 30 minutes.

2. Meanwhile, in a food processor, combine avocado, cucumber, mint, sour cream, lime juice, water, salt, and cumin. Process until nearly smooth. Transfer to a serving bowl.

3. Preheat the grill to medium high. Thread meat on skewers, leaving ¼ inch between pieces. Place skewers on the grill, cover, and grill 10 to 12 minutes for medium rare, turning to brown evenly. Serve steaks with avocado sauce.

TABLE TALK

If you plan to use bamboo skewers, soak them in water while the beef marinates.

Grilled Pork with Nectarines

Grilled nectarines and cherries add a sweet note to lean pork tenderloin.

Yield:	Prep time:	Cook time:	Serving size:
1½ pounds pork and 9 cups salad	10 minutes	8 to 12 minutes	¼ pound pork and 1½ cups salad

Each serving has:				
269 calories	9.3 g total fat	2 g saturated fat	83 mg cholesterol	167 mg sodium
15.5 g carbohydrates	2.1 g fiber	8.2 g sugars	31.4 g protein	

1½ lb. pork tenderloin, cut into ¾-in.-thick slices

4 nectarines, halved and pitted

3 cups sweet cherries, halved and pitted

2 TB. olive oil

2 TB. lemon juice

½ tsp. poppy seeds

¼ tsp. chili powder

¼ tsp. salt

4 cups mixed salad greens

1. Heat the grill to medium. Lightly oil grill. Grill pork slices on the rack of the uncovered grill for 6 minutes, turning once, or until pork is done to an internal temperature of 160°F.

2. Toss nectarines and cherries with oil. Place in the grill basket. Grill 2 minutes per side.

3. In a small bowl, whisk together lemon juice, poppy seeds, chili powder, and salt to make a dressing. Arrange greens, pork, and fruit on 6 serving plates. Drizzle dressing on salads.

TABLE TALK

Poppy seeds give visual interest to this salad and highlight the sweet tastes of the nectarines and cherries.

Brisket with Peppercorns

Peppercorns bring out the flavor of beef brisket that's served with a creamy balsamic vinegar sauce.

Yield:	Prep time:	Cook time:	Serving size:
3 pounds brisket	15 minutes	2 hours 15 minutes	$\frac{1}{4}$ pound brisket and $\frac{1}{12}$ vegetables and sauce

Each serving has:				
259 calories	9.7 g total fat	3.9 g saturated fat	106 g cholesterol	421 mg sodium
3 mg carbohydrates	0 g fiber	1.4 g sugars	37 g protein	

1 TB. olive oil	1 cup reduced-sodium beef broth
3 lb. beef brisket, trimmed of visible fat	1 TB. Worcestershire sauce
1 TB. mixed peppercorns, coarsely crushed	1 TB. *fines herbes,* crushed
3 medium yellow onions, sliced	$\frac{1}{2}$ cup whipping cream
2 (28-oz.) cans crushed tomatoes	3 TB. balsamic vinegar

1. Heat oil in a large, heavy skillet. Add beef brisket to the hot skillet and sprinkle with peppercorns. Brown brisket on both sides in hot oil and then remove from the skillet.

2. Add onions to the skillet. Cook and stir until tender. Add brisket back to the skillet, along with tomatoes, broth, Worcestershire, and fines herbes. Bring to a boil and then reduce heat to a simmer. Spoon some of onion mixture over brisket. Simmer, covered, 3 hours or until brisket is tender.

3. To serve, remove brisket from the skillet. Meanwhile, skim fat from sauce in the skillet. Stir in cream and vinegar. Bring just to boiling. Remove from heat. Slice brisket and top with pan sauces to serve.

DEFINITION

Fines herbes are a mixture of equal amounts of chopped tarragon, chervil, chives, and parsley.

Poultry
Main Dishes

In This Chapter

- A wide variety of chicken recipes
- Eating free-range, drug-free chicken
- Enjoying new taste combinations with poultry
- Adding anti-inflammation ingredients to traditional poultry dishes

Our chicken recipes are quite varied because so many different flavors and ingredients taste great with chicken. Chicken is mild and readily takes on the flavors of sweet ingredients such as fruit, cinnamon, fennel, carrots, and balsamic vinegar. It's equally delicious with savory tastes like onions, garlic, broccoli, mustard, and legumes.

Our recipes call for the low-fat parts of the chicken, usually breast meat, and ignore the fat-laden skin. The recommended cooking methods make the most of chicken's low-fat qualities, using such techniques as grilling and roasting.

Not all chickens are raised equally, so be sure the poultry you purchase is drug free and preferably free range. You'll be reducing the possibility of eating undesirable inflammatory substances.

Each of these 15 recipes is carefully designed to give you delicious and succulent meals. To maintain the anti-inflammatory character of the meals, be sure to eat only the suggested serving amounts. Usually that's about 3 to 4 ounces of chicken meat, which is plenty to stoke your energy and provide adequate amounts of complete protein.

Bon appetit!

Chicken Marengo

Thyme and garlic lend a succulent flavor to chicken with mushrooms and tomatoes.

Yield:	Prep time:	Cook time:	Serving size:
2 pounds chicken and 4 cups vegetables	10 minutes	15 to 20 minutes	4 ounces chicken and $\frac{1}{2}$ cup vegetables

Each serving has:				
260 calories	11.9 g total fat	2.8 g saturated fat	1.1 mg cholesterol	101 mg sodium
3 g carbohydrates	0.9 g fiber	1.7 g sugars	33.8 g protein	

2 TB. olive oil

2 cups white mushrooms, sliced

1 tsp. garlic, minced

1 tsp. dried thyme, crumbled

2 lb. boneless, skinless chicken breasts, cut into 2-in. fingers

1 (14–15 oz.) can whole tomatoes, drained and chopped

2 TB. lemon juice

1. In a large skillet over medium heat, heat oil and sauté mushrooms, garlic, and thyme. Remove from the pan and set aside. Add chicken to the skillet and cook, turning once, until juices run clear, 5 to 10 minutes.

2. Add tomatoes, lemon juice, and mushroom mixture to chicken and simmer for 5 minutes. Serve warm.

TABLE TALK

Chicken Marengo is known as a favorite dish of Napoleon. We modified the original recipe to give you higher anti-inflammatory value with great taste.

Curried Chicken with Cauliflower

Garden vegetables and chicken are lightly cooked in garlic and curry.

Yield:	Prep time:	Cook time:	Serving size:
8 cups	10 minutes	15 minutes	1⅓ cups

Each serving has:				
240 calories	7.5 g total fat	1.8 g saturated fat	52 mg cholesterol	145 mg sodium
21.6 g carbohydrates	3.3 g fiber	7.2 g sugars	24.6 g protein	

2 TB. olive oil

2 tsp. garlic, minced

12 oz. boneless, skinless chicken breasts, chopped

2 tsp. curry powder

4 cups cauliflower, chopped

1 red bell pepper, cored, seeded, and chopped

1 medium yam, unpeeled and cut into 1-in. pieces

3 cups reduced-sodium chicken broth

½ tsp. freshly ground black pepper

1 large bunch green onions, chopped

½ cup fresh cilantro, chopped

1½ cups nonfat plain Greek-style yogurt

1. In a 4-quart saucepan, heat oil and sauté garlic over medium heat for 1 minute. Add chicken and sprinkle with curry powder. When edges of chicken turn white, after about 3 minutes, flip pieces. Cook for 1 to 3 minutes more, until chicken is lightly golden. Add cauliflower, bell pepper, yam, and broth. Bring to a boil, and then reduce heat and simmer for 10 minutes, until cauliflower and yam are tender. Uncover and cook 2 to 3 minutes until sauce thickens.

2. Season with black pepper. Spoon into 6 bowls and top evenly with green onions and cilantro. Finish each bowl with ¼ cup dollop of yogurt.

TABLE TALK

If you want more heat in this curry, add ½ teaspoon cumin with one chopped jalapeño, or 2 teaspoons chili powder.

Baked Chicken Asian Style

Chicken thighs and drumsticks are baked in a flavorful rice vinegar, soy sauce, and ginger sauce and topped with toasted sesame seeds.

Yield:	Prep time:	Cook time:	Serving size:
8 chicken pieces	10 minutes	45-60 minutes	2 chicken pieces

Each serving has:				
381 calories	14.1 g total fat	3.8 g saturated fat	170 mg cholesterol	347 mg sodium
3.2 g carbohydrates	0.7 g fiber	0 g sugars	55.8 g protein	

1 bunch green onions

2 TB. rice vinegar

1 TB. reduced-sodium soy sauce

1 TB. fresh ginger, minced

1 TB. garlic, minced

1 tsp. Asian hot sauce

¼ tsp. Chinese five-spice powder

4 bone-in chicken thighs, skin removed and trimmed

4 chicken drumsticks, skin removed and trimmed

1½ tsp. toasted sesame seeds

1. Preheat oven to 350°F. Coat a 9×13-inch baking dish with cooking spray.

2. Thinly slice half the onion greens; set aside. Mince the onion whites.

3. Whisk onion whites, vinegar, soy sauce, ginger, garlic, hot sauce, and five-spice powder in a large bowl. Add chicken and toss to coat. Arrange chicken in an even layer in the prepared baking dish, meatier sides down. Pour any remaining sauce from the bowl over chicken.

4. Bake, turning once halfway through so the meatier side is up, until a thermometer inserted into the thickest part of the chicken without touching bone registers 165°F, 45 minutes to 1 hour.

5. Transfer chicken to a serving platter and top with any remaining sauce from the baking dish. Sprinkle with sesame seeds and reserved onion greens.

HEALTHY NOTE

Prepared sauces for Asian cooking are usually very high in sodium, so be sure to purchase those with reduced sodium or no sodium for a healthier meal.

Chicken with Pine Nut Tomato Pesto

Sun-dried tomatoes add brightness and sweetness to this baked chicken.

Yield:	Prep time:	Cook time:	Serving size:
4 chicken breasts	10 minutes	30 to 45 minutes	$^2/_3$ chicken breast

Each serving has:				
231 calories	15.9 g total fat	2.5 g saturated fat	50 mg cholesterol	92 mg sodium
4.8 g carbohydrates	1.2 g fiber	0 g sugars	18.1 g protein	

4½ oz. sun-dried tomatoes in oil, drained and chopped	3 TB. olive oil
2 tsp. garlic, minced	4 boneless, skinless chicken breasts, about 1 lb.
6 TB. pine nuts, lightly toasted	

1. Preheat oven to 400°F.

2. To make pesto, place sun-dried tomatoes, garlic, 4 tablespoons pine nuts, and olive oil into a food processor and process until it becomes a coarse paste.

3. Arrange chicken in a large, ovenproof dish or roasting pan. Spread a tablespoon of pesto over each breast.

4. Roast chicken for 30 to 45 minutes, or until tender and juices run clear when a fork is inserted into thickest part of meat.

5. Arrange chicken on a serving platter and sprinkle with remaining 2 tablespoons toasted pine nuts.

TABLE TALK

Store any remaining pesto in an airtight container in the refrigerator for up to 1 week.

Chicken with Lentils

Cumin and coriander lend a Middle Eastern flavor to lentils served with spiced chicken.

Yield:	Prep time:	Cook time:	Serving size:
4 chicken breasts and 2 cups lentils	10 minutes	47 to 57 minutes	½ chicken breast and ¼ cup lentils

Each serving has:				
389 calories	10.8 g total fat	6 g saturated fat	69 mg cholesterol	83 mg sodium
36.5 g carbohydrates	16.7 g fiber	3.8 g sugars	35.4 g protein	

4 (4-oz.) boneless, skinless chicken breasts	1 tsp. coriander powder
1 TB. maple syrup	2 tsp. garlic, minced
1 tsp. ground cinnamon	1 (15-oz.) can lentils, rinsed and drained
2 TB. olive oil	1 TB. butter
½ cup reduced-salt chicken stock	½ cup chopped fresh parsley
2 medium red onions, sliced	¼ tsp. freshly ground black pepper
1 tsp. cumin powder	

1. Preheat oven to 375°F. Arrange chicken in a roasting pan.

2. In a small bowl, whisk together maple syrup, cinnamon, and 1 tablespoon olive oil, and brush over chicken.

3. Pour stock into the roasting pan and tuck onion slices around chicken. Bake uncovered for 35 to 45 minutes.

4. Heat 1 tablespoon olive oil in a skillet over low heat. Add cumin, coriander, and garlic, and cook for 1 to 2 minutes, stirring constantly. Add lentils and cook for 10 minutes, stirring carefully.

5. Remove chicken to a side dish, put roasting pan on stove over medium heat, and bring liquid to a simmer while stirring to combine pan juices and onions. Stir in butter, half of parsley, and pepper.

6. To serve, divide lentils among 4 warmed serving plates. Add one piece chicken to each plate, top with sauce from pan, and sprinkle with remaining parsley. Serve with steamed broccoli or green beans.

Pesto Chicken with Ricotta

A balsamic vinaigrette dresses roasted chicken stuffed with pesto and ricotta.

Yield:	Prep time:	Cook time:	Serving size:
1½ pounds chicken	15 minutes	20 to 30 minutes	4 ounces chicken

Each serving has:				
232 calories	12.2 g total fat	2.2 g saturated fat	72 mg cholesterol	346 mg sodium
2 g carbohydrates	0.5 g fiber	1.7 g sugars	25.8 g protein	

2 TB. pesto sauce	¼ tsp. freshly ground black pepper
4 oz. low-fat ricotta cheese	2 TB. balsamic vinegar
4 (6-oz.) boneless, skinless chicken breasts	1 TB. lemon juice
5 TB. olive oil	¼ cup fresh basil, finely chopped
	¼ tsp. salt

1. Preheat oven to 350°F.

2. Mix pesto and ricotta in a small bowl until well combined. Using a sharp knife, cut a deep slit into the side of each chicken breast to make a pocket. Spoon ricotta mixture into the pockets and reshape chicken breasts to enclose mixture.

3. Brush chicken with 1 tablespoon olive oil and season with pepper. Bake until juices run clear, 20 to 30 minutes.

4. To make vinaigrette, place 4 tablespoons olive oil, balsamic vinegar, lemon juice, basil, and salt in a jar with a screw-top lid. Close the lid and shake the jar to blend.

5. Cut chicken into 6 equal portions. Transfer to 6 serving plates, spoon vinaigrette over chicken, and serve at once.

TABLE TALK

Pesto is traditionally made with fresh basil, garlic, pine nuts, and olive oil.

Chicken with Walnuts

Walnuts, garlic, and Parmesan are flavored with mace and rolled up inside chicken breasts.

Yield:	Prep time:	Cook time:	Serving size:
6 breasts	15 minutes	25 to 30 minutes	1 breast

Each serving has:				
302 calories	5.4 g total fat	1 g saturated fat	67 mg cholesterol	373 mg sodium
9 g carbohydrates	1.3 g fiber	1 g sugars	26.6 g protein	

6 (4-oz.) boneless, skinless chicken breasts

3 slices whole-wheat bread, chopped

2 shallots, finely chopped

2 tsp. garlic, minced

2 TB. finely chopped fresh flat-leaf parsley

2 TB. Parmesan cheese, grated

4 TB. walnuts, finely chopped

¼ tsp. ground mace

¼ tsp. salt

¼ tsp. freshly ground black pepper

Olive oil, for brushing

6 sprigs fresh flat-leaf parsley

1. Place chicken breasts on a wooden cutting board or between 2 sheets of plastic wrap and pound gently with a meat mallet or the side of a rolling pin to flatten.

2. In a food processor, process bread, shallots, garlic, chopped parsley, Parmesan, walnuts, mace, salt, and pepper.

3. Spread bread filling evenly over chicken breasts and roll up. Secure each roll with a wooden toothpick. Brush chicken rolls with oil and grill, turning once, for 25-30 minutes, or until cooked through and tender. Serve at once, garnished with parsley sprigs.

TABLE TALK

These chicken rollups are great served at room temperature for lunchboxes and picnics.

Chicken with Walnut Sauce

Walnut sauce with garlic and yogurt flavor this skillet-cooked chicken.

Yield:	Prep time:	Cook time:	Serving size:
1½ pounds chicken and 2 cups walnut sauce	15 minutes	20 minutes	4 ounces chicken and ⅓ cup walnut sauce

Each serving has:				
433 calories	27.7 g total fat	4.1 g saturated fat	102 mg cholesterol	206 mg sodium
4.8 g carbohydrates	1.5 g fiber	2 g sugars	39.6 g protein	

3 TB. olive oil	1 bay leaf
6 (4-oz.) boneless, skinless chicken breasts	¼ tsp. freshly ground black pepper
2 TB. lemon juice	1 cup walnut pieces
¼ cup dry white wine	2 tsp. garlic, minced
10 oz. reduced-sodium chicken broth	½ cup plain low-fat Greek yogurt

1. Heat oil in a large skillet, add chicken, and brown quickly on all sides.

2. Pour lemon and wine into the skillet and bring to a boil. Add broth, bay leaf, and pepper, and simmer for about 20 minutes, turning once, until chicken is tender. Remove bay leaf.

3. Meanwhile, place walnuts and garlic in a food processor and blend until fairly smooth.

4. When chicken is cooked, transfer to a warmed serving dish and keep warm. Stir walnut mixture and yogurt into the pan juices and heat gently for about 5 minutes until the sauce is quite thick. (Don't boil or sauce will curdle.)

5. Pour walnut sauce over chicken and serve hot.

TABLE TALK

Use any leftover walnut sauce over eggs, grilled meats, or cooked legumes.

Moroccan Chicken Tagine

A delicious combination of chicken, eggplant, chickpeas, and apricots cooked with cumin and mushrooms, and flavored with garlic and cilantro.

Yield:	Prep time:	Cook time:	Serving size:
8 cups	20 minutes	30 minutes	1⅓ cups

Each serving has:				
308 calories	6.7 g total fat	0.9 g saturated fat	33 mg cholesterol	330 mg sodium
38.7 g carbohydrates	11.1 g fiber	8.4 g sugars	23.4 g protein	

1 TB. olive oil

1 medium yellow onion, cut into small wedges

3 garlic cloves, sliced

1 lb. boneless, skinless chicken breast, cut in ½-in. chunks

1 tsp. ground cumin

2 cinnamon sticks

1 TB. whole-wheat flour

1 small eggplant, diced

1 red bell pepper, cored, seeded, and chopped

1 cup white mushrooms, sliced

1 TB. tomato paste

2 cups reduced-sodium chicken broth

1 (15-oz.) can chickpeas, rinsed and drained

¼ cup dried apricots, chopped

¼ tsp. salt

¼ tsp. freshly ground black pepper

1 TB. fresh cilantro, chopped

1. Heat oil in a large pan over medium heat. Add onion and garlic to pan and cook for 3 minutes, stirring frequently. Add chicken, cumin, and cinnamon sticks, and cook, stirring constantly, for another 5 minutes.

2. Sprinkle flour over chicken mixture and cook, stirring constantly, for 2 minutes. Add eggplant, bell pepper, and mushrooms, and cook for 2 minutes, stirring constantly.

3. In a separate bowl, blend tomato paste with broth, and then stir into the pan and bring to a boil. Reduce heat and add chickpeas and apricots. Cover and simmer for 15 to 20 minutes, or until chicken is tender.

4. Season with salt and pepper and serve at once, sprinkled with cilantro.

TABLE TALK

In Morocco, a tagine is both a meat/vegetable stew and an earthenware covered pot used for cooking the stew over an outdoor open-flame stove or oven.

Chicken with Rice and Lemons

Saffron and green olives enhance the flavor of chicken with bell peppers and lemon.

Yield:	Prep time:	Cook time:	Serving size:
1 pound chicken and 6 cups rice/vegetable mixture	20 minutes	65 minutes	4 ounces chicken and 1 cup rice/vegetable mixture

Each serving has:				
388 calories	13.2 g total fat	2.9 g saturated fat	101 mg cholesterol	513 mg sodium
27.8 g carbohydrates	2.2 g fiber	4.5 g sugars	36.7 g protein	

1 TB. olive oil	2 yellow bell peppers, cored, seeded, and cut into chunks
2 tsp. garlic, minced and crushed	1 lemon, cut into 8 wedges
1 large white onion, thinly sliced	$\frac{1}{2}$ cup brown basmati rice
1$\frac{1}{2}$ cups reduced-sodium chicken broth	$\frac{1}{2}$ tsp. freshly ground black pepper
$\frac{1}{2}$ tsp. saffron threads	4 pimento-stuffed green olives
4 (4-oz.) boneless, skinless chicken breasts	

1. Preheat oven to 350°F.

2. Heat oil in a large skillet over low heat. Add garlic and onion, and cook for 1 minute, stirring constantly. Add broth and saffron, and cook over low heat until heated throughout.

3. Place chicken in a large casserole dish with bell peppers, lemons, and rice. Pour broth mixture in the dish, mix well, and season with pepper.

4. Cover and bake for 50 minutes, or until chicken is cooked through and tender. Reduce the oven temperature to 325°F. Add olives to the casserole and cook for an additional 10 minutes.

5. Garnish with lemon wedges and serve immediately. This dish is also delicious served cold.

TABLE TALK

Saffron is a rare and high-priced bright yellow spice. If unavailable, substitute $\frac{1}{2}$ teaspoon turmeric.

Curry Chicken Stir-Fry

Chicken thighs are stir-fried with lime, lemongrass, and peanuts in a Thai-style dish.

Yield:	Prep time:	Cook time:	Serving size:
meat from 6 thighs and 3 cups vegetables	10 minutes	15 minutes	meat from 1 thigh and ¹/₂ cup vegetables

Each serving has:				
384 calories	23.7 g total fat	10.6 g saturated fat	66 mg cholesterol	395 mg sodium
13.8 g carbohydrates	4.2 g fiber	5.9 g sugars	30.3 g protein	

1 TB. olive oil

2 white onions, sliced

2 TB. curry powder

1 cup unsweetened coconut milk

¹/₂ cup water

4 kaffir lime leaves, torn coarsely

1 lemongrass stalk, chopped finely

6 boneless, skinless chicken thighs, chopped into 1-in. pieces

2 TB. reduced-sodium soy sauce

³/₄ cup unsalted peanuts, roasted and chopped

¹/₂ cup fresh pineapple, coarsely chopped

1 small cucumber, peeled, seeded, and thickly sliced

1. Heat oil in a wok and stir-fry onions for 1 minute. Sprinkle with curry and stir-fry for another 1 to 2 minutes.

2. Pour in coconut milk and water. Add lime leaves and lemongrass, and simmer for 1 minute. Add chicken and gradually bring to a boil. Simmer for 8 to 10 minutes until chicken is tender.

3. Stir in soy sauce and let simmer for 1 to 2 minutes. Stir in ¹/₂ cup peanuts, pineapple, and ²/₃ of cucumber slices, and cook for 30 seconds. Serve immediately, sprinkled with remaining peanuts and cucumber.

TABLE TALK

Kaffir lime leaves come from a lime tree native to Southeast Asia. The fruit is used in Lao and Thai curry paste, adding an aromatic and stringent flavor. If they aren't available in your area, you can omit from the recipe.

Chicken Vindaloo

Traditional Indian spices flavor chicken cooked with yams.

Yield:	Prep time:	Cook time:	Serving size:
9 cups	10 minutes	1 hour 8 minutes	1½ cups

Each serving has:				
367 calories	12.6 g total fat	2.7 g saturated fat	87 mg cholesterol	200 mg sodium
31.8 g carbohydrates	5.7 g fiber	4.9 g sugars	31.3 g protein	

1 tsp. ground cumin	3 medium red onions, sliced
1 tsp. ground cinnamon	4 (4-oz.) skinless, boneless chicken breasts, cut into bite-size pieces
2 tsp. mustard powder	
1 tsp. ground coriander	1 lb. yams, peeled and chopped
1 tsp. cayenne pepper	1 lb. canned tomatoes, diced
1 tsp. red chili powder	¼ cup tomato paste
5 TB. red wine vinegar	¼ tsp. salt
2 TB. olive oil	¼ tsp. freshly ground black pepper
8 tsp. garlic, minced	

1. Mix together cumin, cinnamon, mustard powder, coriander, cayenne pepper, and chili powder in a small bowl. Add vinegar and mix well.

2. Heat oil in a large skillet. Add garlic and onions, and cook, stirring, over medium heat for 5 minutes. Add chicken and cook for another 3 minutes, and then add yams, tomatoes, and tomato paste. Stir in spice mixture, season with salt and pepper, and bring to a boil. Lower the heat, cover the pan, and let simmer, stirring occasionally, for 1 hour. Serve.

TABLE TALK

If you prefer, increase the heat of this traditional Indian dish by adding one or two finely diced red or green chili peppers.

Chicken with Prunes and Hazelnuts

Oregano and bay leaf season this dish flavored with prunes and yogurt.

Yield:	Prep time:	Cook time:	Serving size:
6 chicken breasts and 2 cups sauce	10 minutes	35 minutes	1 chicken breast and $\frac{1}{3}$ cup sauce

Each serving has:				
397 calories	13.6 g total fat	3 g saturated fat	102 mg cholesterol	213 mg sodium
34.7 g carbohydrates	4.1 g fiber	20.9 g sugars	35.6 g protein	

1 TB. olive oil	3 TB. balsamic vinegar
6 (4-oz.) boneless, skinless chicken breasts	6 pitted prunes, halved
1 tsp. dried oregano	$\frac{1}{3}$ cup chopped hazelnuts
1 bay leaf	$\frac{1}{4}$ tsp. salt
$\frac{1}{2}$ cup water	$\frac{1}{4}$ tsp. freshly ground black pepper
	$\frac{1}{2}$ cup low-fat Greek yogurt

1. In a large, heavy skillet with a tight-fitting lid, heat oil. Add chicken and cook about 10 minutes, turning once. Add oregano, bay leaf, water, vinegar, prunes, hazelnuts, salt, and pepper.

2. Cover and cook over low heat until chicken is cooked through, about 25 minutes.

3. Remove chicken from the skillet to a serving plate. Stir yogurt into the skillet and heat until blended and warm. Remove bay leaf. Spoon sauce over chicken and serve.

TABLE TALK

Food packaging at the grocery store uses the term "dried plums" in place of "prunes." Don't be confused—in either package, they're delicious in this dish.

Caribbean Chicken

A tangy marinade of garlic, allspice, and black pepper flavors grilled chicken breasts.

Yield:	Prep time:	Cook time:	Serving size:
12 chicken fingers	1 hour plus marinate time	10 to 15 minutes	2 chicken fingers

Each serving has:				
241 calories	10.7 g total fat	2.6 g saturated fat	101 mg cholesterol	195 mg sodium
1.3 g carbohydrates	0 g fiber	0 g sugars	33 g protein	

¼ cup white wine vinegar	1¼ tsp. freshly ground black pepper
1 TB. fresh ginger, minced	¼ tsp. salt
4 cloves garlic, minced	4 (6-oz.) boneless, skinless chicken breast halves, cut into 3 fingers each
1½ TB. olive oil	
1 TB. allspice	

1. In a large bowl, combine vinegar, ginger, garlic, oil, allspice, pepper, and salt. Add chicken and turn to coat on all sides. Cover and refrigerate for up to 1 hour.

2. Preheat the grill to medium.

3. Lift chicken from marinade and place chicken on the grill. Discard marinade. Grill 4 to 6 inches from heat, turning once, for 10 to 15 minutes or until cooked through.

TABLE TALK

You can bake the marinated chicken in a 350°F oven for 20 to 30 minutes, basting the chicken with marinade several times while it bakes.

Turkey Steaks with Pears

Turkey is rubbed with sage, served with spinach and pears, and topped with blue cheese crumbles.

Yield:	Prep time:	Cook time:	Serving size:
4 turkey steaks and 2 cups sides and topping	10 minutes	21 to 23 minutes	1 turkey steak and $\frac{1}{2}$ cup sides and topping

Each serving has:				
241 calories	11 g total fat	3.2 g saturated fat	76 mg cholesterol	167 mg sodium
3.6 g carbohydrates	1.4 g fiber	2.4 g sugars	29.8 g protein	

2 turkey breast tenderloins (1¼ lb.)	6 oz. baby spinach
1 tsp. dried sage	1 large pear, cored and thinly sliced
2 TB. olive oil	¼ cup crumbled blue cheese

1. Split turkey tenderloins to make 4 steaks. Rub turkey with sage.

2. In a very large skillet, heat 1 tablespoon olive oil and cook steaks over medium-high heat for 14 to 16 minutes, turning once. Meat should register 170°F on a meat thermometer. Remove from the skillet. Lower heat to medium.

3. Add spinach to the skillet and stir just until wilted.

4. In a small skillet, cook pear slices in 1 tablespoon olive oil over medium heat for 5 minutes or until slightly browned.

5. Serve turkey with spinach and pears. Crumble blue cheese over all.

TABLE TALK

Purchase blue cheese that's already crumbled or crumble your own from a block of cheese.

Seafood Main Dishes

In This Chapter

- Enjoying the bounty of sea and stream
- Gaining the benefits of eating fish rich in omega-3
- Cooking for seafood tenderness and taste
- Adding succulent vegetables and spices to seafood

Fish is an excellent choice for eating to lower inflammation. It contains lean and tasty complete protein, and it's easy to prepare. Cold-water fish, such as salmon, contain high amounts of omega-3 essential fatty acids that are known to reduce inflammation, soothe aching joints and ligaments, and uplift moods.

But purchasing fresh, frozen, canned, or packaged fish is challenging. As best you can, purchase wild fish that is mercury free. Wild fish is generally healthier to eat than farmed fish. Be sure to ask for details about the fish before you purchase it.

Canned salmon is safe to eat up to four times a month. It's canned on ship immediately after it's caught.

Because the information on fish safety changes, you can learn more about which fish to purchase at websites such as intraspec.ca/fish.php and www.organicconsumers.org/Toxic/safe-fish.cfm.

When you've selected the best and healthiest fish and you're ready to cook, check out the recipes in this chapter and enjoy every healthful bite.

Halibut with Fennel

Sun-dried tomatoes, fennel, and kalamata olives add a Mediterranean flavor to the halibut.

Yield:	Prep time:	Cook time:	Serving size:
4 packets	10 minutes	12 to 14 minutes	1 packet

Each serving has:				
295 calories	8.6 g total fat	1.2 g saturated fat	58 mg cholesterol	177 mg sodium
14.2 g carbohydrates	4.6 g fiber	5.8 g sugars	40.6 g protein	

4 (5-oz.) halibut fillets

1 TB. olive oil

1 tsp. garlic powder

1 tsp. red pepper flakes

6 sun-dried tomatoes, chopped

1 small red onion, thinly sliced

1 fennel bulb, cored and thinly sliced

4 kalamata or other black olives, drained, pitted, and sliced

1. Preheat oven to 400°F.

2. Tear off 4 pieces of foil to form squares. Place one fillet in the center of each square.

3. Drizzle each fillet with oil, and season with garlic powder and red pepper. Sprinkle sun-dried tomatoes evenly over top. Arrange onion slices over fish, and top with fennel and olives.

4. Fold aluminum foil around fish to make 4 enclosed packets, keeping seam at the tops of the packets.

5. Place the packets on a large baking sheet in the oven and cook for 12 to 14 minutes, depending on thickness of fish. Remove the baking dish from the oven and place on a serving dish. Carefully unfold foil to allow steam to escape. Serve immediately.

TABLE TALK

Kalamata olives have a stronger taste than regular black olives. They are named after the city of Kalamata, Greece, and are a staple of Greek cooking.

Mediterranean Cod

Pine nuts, raisins, and cocoa add exotic flavor to baked cod.

Yield:	Prep time:	Cook time:	Serving size:
2¼ pounds cod	10 minutes	15 to 25 minutes	⅓ pound cod

Each serving has:				
284 calories	9.9 g total fat	1.2 g saturated fat	94 mg cholesterol	213 mg sodium
7.7 g carbohydrates	0.8 g fiber	4.8 g sugars	40 g protein	

2¼ lb. cod

2 TB. olive oil

1 white medium onion, thinly sliced

¼ cup pine nuts

¼ cup raisins

1 TB. lemon zest

½ tsp. cinnamon

1 tsp. unsweetened cocoa powder

¼ tsp. freshly ground black pepper

½ cup reduced-sodium vegetable broth

1 tsp. cider vinegar

1 bay leaf

1. Preheat oven to 350°F.

2. Place cod in an oiled baking dish. Drizzle cod with oil. Top with onion, pine nuts, raisins, lemon zest, cinnamon, cocoa powder, and pepper.

3. Pour broth and vinegar around fish. Add bay leaf. Place fish in the oven and bake for 15 to 25 minutes, until fish flakes when gently separated with a fork. Remove bay leaf and serve.

TABLE TALK

The cocoa powder adds a rich, slightly bitter taste that accents the sweetness of the raisins and pine nuts.

Swordfish Steaks

Asiago cheese lightly flavors swordfish steaks tipped with capers and parsley.

Yield:	Prep time:	Cook time:	Serving size:
1¾ pounds swordfish	12 minutes	10 to 20 minutes	7 ounces swordfish

Each serving has:				
353 calories	14.3 g total fat	4.2 g saturated fat	82 mg cholesterol	423 mg sodium
9.9 g carbohydrates	0.7 g fiber	0.9 g sugars	43.1 g protein	

1¾ lb. swordfish, thinly sliced	1 TB. capers, drained and chopped
½ cup stone-ground breadcrumbs	2 TB. asiago cheese, grated
¼ tsp. freshly ground black pepper	3 TB. olive oil
2 TB. fresh parsley, finely chopped	

1. Gently flatten swordfish steaks using a meat mallet, and cut into 4 pieces. Season breadcrumbs with pepper and chopped parsley. Mix in capers and cheese. Coat swordfish steaks with breadcrumb mixture.

2. Heat oil in a large nonstick skillet over medium heat. Place steaks in the skillet and cook for 15 to 20 minutes, turning once after 8 minutes. Fish is done when flesh flakes and can be separated with a fork. Serve immediately.

HEALTHY NOTE

Add a green salad to this fish meal for nutritional balance.

Grouper with Mushrooms

White wine, garlic, and almonds add European flavor to this fish sautéed with mushrooms.

Yield:	Prep time:	Cook time:	Serving size:
1¾ pounds grouper and 2 cups vegetables	15 minutes	16 minutes	⅖ pound grouper and ½ cup vegetables

Each serving has:				
342 calories	9.7 g total fat	1.4 g saturated fat	93 mg cholesterol	260 mg sodium
7.3 g carbohydrates	2.2 g fiber	3.1 g sugars	52.3 g protein	

1 small white onion, thinly sliced	¼ tsp. salt
2 tsp. garlic, minced	¼ tsp. freshly ground black pepper
1 TB. olive oil	½ cup water
1¾ lb. grouper fillets, cut in 4 portions	1 bay leaf
¼ cup white wine	1 cup white mushrooms, sliced
2 medium tomatoes, cut in wedges	¼ cup fresh parsley
	2 TB. almonds, slivered

1. In a large nonstick skillet, sauté onion and garlic in oil for 1 minute.

2. Add fillets and cook gently for 5 minutes, turning once. Add white wine and simmer until it evaporates.

3. Add tomatoes to skillet. Season with salt and pepper, and add water, bay leaf, and mushrooms. Cover and cook 5 minutes. Remove lid and cook for another 5 minutes. Remove bay leaf.

4. Place fish and vegetables on a serving platter. Sprinkle with parsley and almonds. Serve immediately.

HEALTHY NOTE

Use an up-to-date nonstick skillet that's coated in enamel or another nonreactive surface. Take some time to go through your cabinets and toss any older nonstick pans that are scratched or coated with Teflon.

Salmon with Lemon

Salmon is gently sautéed with garlic and a hint of lemon.

Yield:	Prep time:	Cook time:	Serving size:
4 slices salmon	5 minutes	16 minutes	1 slice salmon

Each serving has:				
482 calories	31.5 g total fat	6.8 g saturated fat	125 mg cholesterol	124 mg sodium
3.2 g carbohydrates	1.2 g fiber	0 g sugars	44.4 g protein	

2 TB. olive oil	3 TB. lemon juice
2 garlic cloves	¼ cup fresh parsley, chopped
1¾ lb. salmon, cut into 4 slices	2 TB. fresh oregano, chopped

1. Heat oil in a large nonstick skillet. Add garlic cloves and sauté for 1 to 2 minutes. Add salmon and cook for 8 minutes on one side. Turn salmon and cook for another 4 minutes or until fish is almost done.

2. Add lemon juice and cook for 2 to 4 more minutes, until fish is cooked throughout. Add parsley and oregano. Serve immediately.

HEALTHY NOTE

The salmon contains the essential omega-3 fatty acids you need to reduce inflammation and improve overall cardiovascular health.

Monkfish in Leek Sauce

Chili adds zing to monkfish cooked with olives and parsley.

Yield:	Prep time:	Cook time:	Serving size:
4 fillets	15 minutes	25 minutes	1 fillet plus ¼ sauce

Each serving has:				
340 calories	12.9 g total fat	1.2 g saturated fat	68 mg cholesterol	216 mg sodium
11.2 g carbohydrates	2.6 g fiber	4.2 g sugars	44.9 g protein	

2 leeks, sliced	½ cup water
2 TB. olive oil	2 lb. monkfish, cut into 4 fillets
¼ tsp. chili powder	½ cup black olives
3 medium tomatoes, cut in wedges	¼ tsp. freshly ground black pepper
¼ cup fresh parsley, chopped	

1. In a large skillet over medium heat, sauté leeks in oil. Add chili powder, tomatoes, parsley, and water, and bring to a boil.

2. Add monkfish and olives to skillet. Reduce heat and simmer, covered, for 15 minutes. Sprinkle with pepper before serving.

TABLE TALK

Monkfish is a strong-bodied fish reminiscent of lobster.

Trout with Cranberries

Cranberries add tang and sweetness to this savory dish.

Yield:	Prep time:	Cook time:	Serving size:
2 pounds trout and 2 cups vegetables with sauce	15 minutes	15 minutes	$\frac{1}{3}$ pound trout and $\frac{1}{3}$ cup vegetables with sauce

Each serving has:				
347 calories	17.4 g total fat	2.9 g saturated fat	112 mg cholesterol	215 mg sodium
4.8 g carbohydrates	0.6 g fiber	3.3 g sugars	40.6 g protein	

1 cup celery, chopped	1 TB. white wine vinegar
$\frac{1}{4}$ cup white onion, chopped	$1\frac{1}{4}$ cups water
$\frac{1}{2}$ tsp. dried sage	3 TB. dried cranberries, soaked in hot water and drained
1 tsp. dried rosemary	$\frac{1}{4}$ tsp. salt
1 tsp. garlic, minced	$\frac{1}{4}$ tsp. freshly ground black pepper
2 TB. olive oil	
2 lb. trout, cut into 6 pieces	

1. In a large skillet over medium heat, sauté celery, onion, sage, rosemary, and garlic in the olive oil.

2. Place trout on top of vegetables in the skillet and add vinegar, water, cranberries, salt, and pepper. Cover and cook 10 minutes. Remove lid and continue cooking until trout is done, about 5 minutes.

3. Place trout portions on 6 plates. Divide vegetables and sauce equally among plates.

TABLE TALK

The small amount of vinegar in this recipe gives it the taste of having been cooked in wine, but saves you the calories and expense.

Teriyaki Salmon with Pineapple

Grilled salmon takes on the Asian flavors of soy sauce and fresh pineapple.

Yield:	Prep time:	Cook time:	Serving size:
4 steaks	5 minutes plus 1½ hours marinate time	10 minutes	1 steak and 1 pineapple ring

Each serving has:				
453 calories	28.1 g total fat	5.2 g saturated fat	107 mg cholesterol	371 mg sodium
10.2 g carbohydrates	1.1 g fiber	6.1 g sugars	38.6 g protein	

¼ cup olive oil	1 tsp. ground ginger
¼ cup lemon juice	1 tsp. garlic, minced
¼ cup reduced-sodium soy sauce	4 (6-oz.) salmon steaks
1 tsp. ground mustard	4 fresh pineapple rings, ½ in. thick

1. In a large resealable plastic bag (or shallow glass container), mix together olive oil, lemon juice, soy sauce, mustard, ginger, and garlic. Set aside half of marinade for basting, and refrigerate.

2. Add salmon to marinade in bag. Seal the bag and refrigerate for 1½ hours, turning once. Drain and discard marinade.

3. Heat the grill over medium heat. Place salmon and pineapple rings on the grill and cook for 5 minutes. Brush salmon with reserved marinade. Turn both salmon and pineapple, and broil for 5 minutes or until fish flakes easily with a fork. Brush salmon with marinade.

4. Serve each salmon fillet with a pineapple ring.

TABLE TALK

Grilling the pineapple brings out the sweetness and is a perfect complement to the tangy taste of the teriyaki.

Salmon Tacos with Avocado Sauce

Chipotle chilies give south-of-the border flavor to tacos.

Yield:	Prep time:	Cook time:	Serving size:
8 tacos	25 minutes	25 minutes	1 taco

Each serving has:				
422 calories	23.7 g total fat	4.3 g saturated fat	63 mg cholesterol	98 mg sodium
27.5 g carbohydrates	7.6 g fiber	4.1 g sugars	27.2 g protein	

4 chipotle chilies

1½ TB. olive oil

1 small white onion, chopped finely

2 tsp. garlic, minced

⅓ cup fresh oregano, coarsely chopped

3 TB. tomato paste

3 TB. water

4 (7-oz.) salmon steaks

2 cups frozen corn, thawed

2 small avocados, peeled, pit removed, and chopped

½ cup low-fat plain yogurt

¼ cup fresh cilantro, coarsely chopped

1½ TB. lime juice

8 large flour tortillas

2 limes, cut into wedges

1. Place chilies in a small heatproof bowl of boiling water. Let stand 15 minutes. Drain and chop coarsely.

2. Heat oil in a large skillet over medium heat. Cook onion and garlic, stirring, until onion softens. Stir in chilies, oregano, tomato paste, and water. Bring to a boil. Remove from heat. Place in a food processor and pulse until mixture forms a thick paste.

3. Place fish in single layer in a large dish. Pat chili paste into both sides of fish.

4. Steam corn in a vegetable steamer for 5 minutes. Place fish in the skillet and cook on medium heat until browned on both sides and cooked to desired temperature, about 15 minutes. Cut salmon into 8 equal pieces.

5. In a small bowl, mash together avocado and yogurt to form a thick mixture. Stir in cilantro and lime juice.

6. Divide fish, corn, avocado cream, and tortillas among 8 serving plates. Serve with lime wedges.

Tilapia with Spinach and Peppers

Feta cheese and spinach top this baked tilapia.

Yield:	Prep time:	Cook time:	Serving size:
4 fillets plus 2 cups salad	8 minutes	20 to 25 minutes	1 fillet and ½ cup salad

Each serving has:				
266 calories	10.4 g total fat	2.8 g saturated fat	77 mg cholesterol	289 mg sodium
8.8 g carbohydrates	2.1 g fiber	3 g sugars	31.8 g protein	

4 (5-oz.) tilapia fillets	4 TB. lemon juice
2 red bell peppers, cored, seeded, and coarsely chopped	2 shallots, diced
2 cloves garlic, thinly sliced	2 TB. olive oil
2 TB. fresh parsley, chopped	4 cups baby spinach
	½ cup low-fat feta cheese

1. Preheat the oven to 350°F. Place fillets and bell peppers in a glass baking dish. Sprinkle garlic, parsley, and lemon juice over top. Cover with foil and bake for 15 to 20 minutes, until fish is opaque and flakes easily with a fork.

2. In a medium skillet over medium-high heat, sauté shallots in oil for 1 minute. Reduce heat to medium and add spinach, cooking until wilted, about 5 minutes. Stir in feta and heat until melted.

3. To serve, place ¾ cup spinach-feta mixture on each plate and top with 1 fillet and peppers.

Variation: If you are sensitive or allergic to dairy products, omit the feta cheese. You can substitute sliced almonds or another vegetable, such as corn or peas.

HEALTHY NOTE

Other leaf vegetables that can add anti-inflammation properties to tilapia are red kale, kale, beet greens, and collard greens.

Salmon with Coriander

Coriander adds sweet Moroccan flavor to baked salmon served with rice and kale.

Yield:	Prep time:	Cook time:	Serving size:
4 fillets, 2 cups rice, 4 cups kale	20 minutes	11 to 13 minutes	1 fillet, $\frac{1}{2}$ cup rice, 1 cup kale

Each serving has:				
439 calories	17.8 g total fat	3.2 g saturated fat	71 mg cholesterol	447 mg sodium
39.5 g carbohydrates	2.8 g fiber	2.4 g sugars	34.2 g protein	

1 cup brown and wild rice blend

1 TB. ground coriander

2 TB. lemon juice

3 tsp. garlic, minced

2 tsp. olive oil

4 (4-oz.) boneless, skinless salmon fillets

12 cups chopped kale stems and leaves (about 1 bunch)

2 TB. water

$\frac{1}{4}$ tsp. salt

$\frac{1}{4}$ tsp. freshly ground black pepper

1. Prepare rice according to package directions. Remove from heat.

2. Preheat oven to 400°F. In a small bowl, combine coriander, 1 tablespoon lemon juice, 2 teaspoons garlic, and 1 teaspoon oil. Rub mixture onto salmon fillets. Transfer salmon to a baking pan and bake for 8 to 10 minutes or until cooked through and the salmon flakes easily with a fork.

3. Meanwhile, in a large nonstick skillet, heat remaining 1 teaspoon oil on medium-high heat. Add half of kale, remaining 1 teaspoon garlic, and water. Cook, stirring, until kale begins to wilt, about 1 minute.

4. Stir in remaining kale and cook, stirring, for 2 minutes. Add salt, pepper, and remaining 1 tablespoon lemon juice. Stir. Divide rice and kale among 4 plates. Top with salmon fillets.

Variation: You can substitute beet greens or Swiss chard for the kale in this recipe.

TABLE TALK

Coriander seeds are the dried seeds of the cilantro plant. You can purchase the seeds whole or ground.

Shrimp with Green Apples

Wasabi-dressed shrimp tops a salad of green apples, papaya, cucumber, and watercress prepared with an Asian-style flavor.

Yield:	Prep time:	Cook time:	Serving size:
2 pounds shrimp and 6 cups salad	15 minutes	None	1/3 cup shrimp and 1 cup salad

Each serving has:				
279 calories	9.5 g total fat	1.3 g saturated fat	216 mg cholesterol	211 mg sodium
21.1 g carbohydrates	3.4 g fiber	11.4 g sugars	30.6 g protein	

3 TB. apple cider vinegar	2 small green apples, cored, sliced into wedges, then sliced thinly
1 tsp. wasabi paste	
1 tsp. garlic, minced	1 small papaya (about 1¼ lb.), peeled, seeds removed, and diced
1½ TB. lemon juice	
¼ cup olive oil	
2 lb. large shrimp, cooked	2 cucumbers, diced
1 small *daikon*	6 cups watercress, trimmed

1. In a small bowl, whisk together vinegar, wasabi, garlic, lemon juice, and oil to make wasabi dressing.

2. Peel and devein shrimp, leaving tails intact.

3. Slice daikon thinly, and then cut slices into matchstick-size pieces. Place in large bowl with apples, papaya, cucumbers, and wasabi dressing. Toss gently to combine.

4. Divide watercress among 6 serving plates. Top with daikon salad and then shrimp.

DEFINITION

Daikon is a form of radish that's white and shaped like a carrot. It's often used in Asian cooking.

Tarragon Sole

Peppery tarragon adds flavor to baked sole fillets.

Yield:	Prep time:	Cook time:	Serving size:
6 fillets	15 minutes	5 to 8 minutes	1 fillet

Each serving has:				
256 calories	8 g total fat	1.5 g saturated fat	112 mg cholesterol	360 mg sodium
13.1 g carbohydrates	0.8 g fiber	1.2 g sugars	30.9 g protein	

6 (4-oz. each) sole fillets

1 large egg

1 TB. water

1 cup whole-wheat panko
   breadcrumbs

1 tsp. tarragon

¼ tsp. salt

¼ tsp. freshly ground black pepper

2 TB. olive oil

1 TB. butter, melted

Lemon wedges

1. Preheat the oven to 350°F. Lightly oil a baking dish large enough to hold fillets in a single layer. Dry sole fillets on paper towels.

2. In a shallow bowl, beat egg with water. In another shallow bowl, mix together panko, tarragon, salt, and pepper.

3. Dip sole in egg and then coat with crumb mixture, patting it on to adhere. Place sole fillets in the baking dish in a single layer.

4. Drizzle oil and butter over fish. Bake on the upper rack of the oven for 5 to 8 minutes, depending on thickness of fish, or until fish just flakes when tested with a fork and the crust is golden brown. Serve with lemon wedges.

TABLE TALK

Tarragon is a light, peppery herb that adds special flavor to homemade mayonnaise and grilled chicken and fish.

Almond Catfish with Mustard

Dijon mustard adds tang and zest to baked catfish.

Yield:	Prep time:	Cook time:	Serving size:
1½ pounds catfish	10 minutes	10 to 15 minutes	6 ounces catfish

Each serving has:			
317 calories	20.5 g total fat	3.8 g saturated fat	84 mg cholesterol	189 mg sodium
3.2 g carbohydrates	1.7 g fiber	0.6 g sugars	29.3 g protein	

4 (6-oz.) catfish fillets	2 tsp. lemon juice
¼ tsp. freshly ground black pepper	1 TB. butter
2 TB. Dijon mustard	½ cup almonds, slivered

1. Preheat the oven to 425°F. Lightly spray a rimmed baking sheet with olive oil.

2. Place fillets on the baking sheet and sprinkle with pepper.

3. In a small bowl, stir together mustard and lemon juice. Spread mixture over tops of fish fillets.

4. In a small skillet, melt butter over medium heat. Add almonds and toss to combine. Spread almond mixture over fish.

5. Bake for 10 to 15 minutes, or until top is golden brown and flesh flakes when tested with a fork.

TABLE TALK

If you prefer not to heat up the house by using the oven, you can pan-fry the catfish using the ingredients in this recipe. You'll need to turn the fish once while it cooks.

Mahi Mahi with Coconut and Salsa

Coconut and lime lend an island flavor to baked mahi mahi.

Yield:	Prep time:	Cook time:	Serving size:
16 pieces fish and 3 cups salsa	15 minutes	15 minutes	4 pieces fish and ¾ cup salsa

Each serving has:				
362 calories	9.9 g total fat	3.7 g saturated fat	197 mg cholesterol	439 mg sodium
28.5 g carbohydrates	3.5 g fiber	7.1 g sugars	37.9 g protein	

1 large egg

1 TB. water

1 cup plain dried whole-wheat breadcrumbs

⅓ cup unsweetened shredded coconut

1½ lb. mahi mahi steaks, cut into 16 chunks

¼ tsp. freshly ground black pepper

1 papaya, peeled, seeds removed, and finely chopped

¼ cup red bell pepper, cored, seeded, and minced

2 green onions, thinly sliced

2 tsp. lime juice

1. Preheat oven to 375°F.

2. In a shallow bowl, beat egg and water. In another shallow bowl, combine breadcrumbs and coconut.

3. Sprinkle fish with black pepper. Dip fish in egg and then in the breadcrumb mixture until well coated. Pat to adhere.

4. Place fish on a nonstick baking dish. Bake for 15 minutes, or until crumbs are crisp and fish chunks can be easily pierced with the tip of a knife.

5. Meanwhile, in a medium bowl combine papaya, bell pepper, onions, and lime juice to make salsa. Serve fish with salsa on the side.

HEALTHY NOTE

The fruit salsa in this recipe combines the sweet taste of papaya and red bell peppers with the bitter, acid taste of onions and the sour taste of lime juice. Add to that the salty and protein taste of the fish, and it's a combination that satisfies all your taste buds.

Halibut with Beets and Cucumbers

Colorful beets tossed with cucumber yogurt dressing brighten sautéed halibut.

Yield:	Prep time:	Cook time:	Serving size:
4 fillets plus 10 cups vegetables	15 minutes	45 to 50 minutes	1 fillet and 2½ cups vegetables

Each serving has:				
366 calories	12.1 g total fat	1.9 g saturated fat	66 mg cholesterol	221 mg sodium
17.1 g carbohydrates	3.5 g fiber	13 g sugars	46.6 g protein	

1 lb. (3 to 4 medium) beets, trimmed and quartered

2 TB. olive oil

¼ tsp. freshly ground black pepper

6 cups Romaine lettuce, torn in pieces

2 cups cucumber, diced

⅓ cup plain low-fat yogurt

1 TB. dill, snipped, or 1 tsp. dried

Pinch of salt

4 halibut fillets (6-oz. each)

1. Preheat the oven to 425°F. Line an ovenproof skillet with foil. Place beets on the foil, drizzle with 1 tablespoon olive oil, and sprinkle with pepper. Seal with more foil and roast for 35 to 40 minutes, until tender. When cool enough to handle, peel and slice.

2. Arrange romaine on 4 dinner plates. Top with the beets and set aside.

3. Toss cucumber with yogurt, half the dill, and salt. Set aside.

4. Heat 1 tablespoon of oil in a large nonstick skillet over medium heat. Place halibut in the skillet and cook for 5 minutes. Turn and cook until the fish just flakes when tested with a fork, about 5 minutes longer. Transfer fish to the serving plates with the beets.

5. Divide cucumber mixture into 4 portions and place beside halibut on plates. Serve.

TABLE TALK

When you're out of fresh herbs, use the ratio of 3:1 for substituting dried herbs. So 1 tablespoon of fresh herbs equals 1 teaspoon dried.

Catfish with Rosemary

Simple catfish is pan-fried with fragrant rosemary sprigs.

Yield:	Prep time:	Cook time:	Serving size:
2 pounds catfish	5 minutes	12 minutes	⅓ pound catfish

Each serving has:			
216 calories	12.9 g total fat	2.6 g saturated fat	73 mg cholesterol	85 mg sodium
0 g carbohydrates	0 g fiber	0 g sugars	23.5 g protein	

1 tsp. olive oil	2 lb. catfish fillets, cut in 6 portions
1 tsp. butter	12 sprigs fresh rosemary

1. In a large nonstick skillet, heat oil and butter over medium heat. Add catfish pieces and rosemary, and cook for 6 minutes. Turn fish and cook 6 minutes until flesh flakes when tested with a fork.

2. Serve with rosemary sprigs on the fish.

HEALTHY NOTE

Be sure to use a nonstick pan with this recipe. The pan lets you reduce the amount of butter you need for cooking, yet the smaller amount lets you enjoy the wonderful flavor of butter.

Salmon Burgers

Quick-cooking salmon cakes are flavored with celery and paprika.

Yield:	Prep time:	Cook time:	Serving size:
4 cakes	10 minutes	23 minutes	1 cake

Each serving has:				
257 calories	12 g total fat	1.6 g saturated fat	53 mg cholesterol	281 mg sodium
13.3 g carbohydrates	1.2 g fiber	2.1 g sugars	22.7 g protein	

2 TB. olive oil	¼ cup celery, chopped
1 small yellow or white onion, minced	3 TB. low-fat mayonnaise
2 cups flaked cooked salmon	1 tsp. smoked paprika
½ cup soft whole-grain breadcrumbs	Lemon wedges

1. In a medium skillet, heat 1 tablespoon oil over medium heat. Add onion and cook, stirring occasionally, until golden brown, about 15 minutes.

2. Transfer onion to a bowl and stir in salmon, breadcrumbs, celery, mayonnaise, and paprika. Form into 4 patties.

3. In a large nonstick skillet, heat remaining 1 tablespoon oil over medium heat. Add salmon cakes and cook until golden brown and cooked through, about 4 minutes per side. Serve with lemon wedges.

TABLE TALK

Making fish cakes is a great way to use leftover fish. You can also use canned salmon in this recipe.

Traditional Crab Cakes

Spicy crab cakes contain bell peppers for crunch and flavor.

Yield:	Prep time:	Cook time:	Serving size:
12 crab cakes	15 minutes	15 minutes	1 crab cake

Each serving has:				
160 calories	6.3 g total fat	1.9 g saturated fat	98 mg cholesterol	411 mg sodium
7.6 g carbohydrates	0.6 g fiber	2.9 g sugars	16.9 g protein	

2 TB. butter	$\frac{1}{2}$ tsp. Worcestershire sauce
$\frac{1}{2}$ cup red bell pepper, minced	6 drops hot pepper sauce
$\frac{1}{2}$ cup green bell pepper, minced	1 large egg
3 green onions, minced	2 lb. lump crabmeat, picked over to remove any cartilage
$\frac{3}{4}$ cup soft stone-ground breadcrumbs	2 TB. olive oil

1. In a large nonstick skillet, melt butter over low heat. Add bell peppers and onions, and cook until peppers are soft, about 5 minutes.

2. Transfer pepper and onion mixture to a bowl and stir in breadcrumbs. Stir in Worcestershire sauce, hot sauce, and egg, until well combined. Gently fold in the crabmeat.

3. With wet hands, form mixture into 12 balls, and then flatten each slightly with the palm of your hand.

4. In the skillet, heat olive oil. Sauté 4 to 6 crab cakes at a time, turning gently with a spatula, until browned on both sides, about 10 minutes. Drain on paper towels.

HEALTHY NOTE

Be sure to use real, not imitation, crab. Imitation crab contains almost double the amount of dietary sodium—a food product to avoid.

Grilled Ancho Salmon with Fries

Yam fries are served with spicy salmon fillets.

Yield:		Prep time:	Cook time:	Serving size:
4 fillets and 4 cups fries		15 minutes	18 to 22 minutes	1 fillet and 1 cup fries

Each serving has:

485 calories	24.5 g total fat	4.5 g saturated fat	89 mg cholesterol	244 mg sodium
31.4 g carbohydrates	4.6 g fiber	0.6 g sugars	33.1 g protein	

¼ tsp. salt	2 TB. olive oil
1 tsp. ground cumin	4 (5-oz.) skinless salmon fillets
1 tsp. ground ancho chili pepper or chili powder	2 TB. fresh cilantro, chopped
2 medium yams, cut in half lengthwise and then into ¼-in. slices	

1. Preheat broiler. In a large bowl, combine salt, cumin, and chili pepper. Reserve half the spices for salmon.

2. Add yams to the bowl. Drizzle with 1 tablespoon olive oil and toss to distribute oil and spices evenly. Place yam slices on a rimmed baking sheet. Broil 4 inches from heat for 10 minutes or until tender, turning once midway through cooking.

3. Sprinkle salmon with reserved spice mixture. In a large nonstick skillet, cook fish in 1 tablespoon hot oil over medium heat for 8 to 12 minutes or until fish flakes when tested with fork, turning once midway through cooking.

4. Place salmon fillets on 4 serving plates. Divide potatoes equally and add to plates. Garnish with cilantro.

TABLE TALK

Serve this entrée with a light garden salad or simple green vegetable to provide contrast to the spicy salmon and fries.

Parmesan-Crusted Tilapia

Parmesan cheese adds flavor to tilapia that's served on a bed of carrots and salad greens.

Yield:	Prep time:	Cook time:	Serving size:
4 fillets and 7 cups vegetables	10 minutes	9 to 11 minutes	1 fillet and 1¾ cups vegetables

Each serving has:				
235 calories	6.5 g total fat	3.6 g saturated fat	96 mg cholesterol	386 mg sodium
10.1 g carbohydrates	3 g fiber	5.1 g sugars	35.4 g protein	

4 (6-oz.) tilapia fillets	3 cups carrots, julienned
¼ tsp. salt	1 TB. butter
¼ tsp. freshly ground black pepper	¾ tsp. ground ginger
¼ cup Parmesan cheese, finely shredded	4 cups mixed fresh salad greens

1. Preheat oven to 450°F.

2. Lightly coat a baking sheet with nonstick cooking spray. Rinse fish and pat dry.

3. Place fish on the baking sheet. Season with salt and pepper. Sprinkle cheese on fish. Bake, uncovered, 4 to 6 minutes for each ½-inch thickness of fish, until fish flakes easily when tested with a fork.

4. Meanwhile, in a vegetable steamer, cook carrots for 5 minutes. Remove to serving bowl. Stir in butter and ginger. Serve fish and carrots next to the greens on individual plates.

HEALTHY NOTE

This recipe gives you a meal with balanced amounts of complete protein, fat, and carbohydrates.

Vegetarian Main Dishes

In This Chapter

- Satisfying recipes with delicious seasonings
- Legumes, burgers, and portobello mushroom entrées
- Lean cooking techniques
- Versatility with your favorite vegetarian foods

Whether or not you prefer to eat only vegetarian meals, you'll enjoy the variety of our meatless entrées. Most recipes offer you a balanced amount of vegetable protein. If you enjoy adding an egg, cheese, or tofu to the meals, you'll find plenty of opportunities.

Because cooking legumes can literally take hours, the recipes often call for canned beans. If you prefer to forgo the convenience factor, you can cook the beans. Remember to soak them in water overnight to soften, then boil and simmer the following day.

If you have difficulty digesting the starch in the beans, you can take a digestive aid supplement especially for beans. The most common product is Bean-O, but you can find other brands at the grocery or health-food store.

Vegetarian cuisine is notably low in saturated fat and cholesterol, so our recipes call for good fats such as olive oil or avocado.

If you aren't familiar with vegetarian cuisine, go ahead and cook up a recipe for a family dinner. You may just get plenty of raves.

Curried Chickpeas

Garbanzo beans are slow cooked, then seasoned with curry, onion, garlic, and collard greens.

Yield:	Prep time:	Cook time:	Serving size:
12 cups	20 minutes	3 to 10 hours	1⅕ cups

Each serving has:				
470 calories	7.3 g total fat	1 g saturated fat	1 mg cholesterol	229 mg sodium
82.4 g carbohydrates	18.7 g fiber	13.5 g sugars	21.6 g protein	

2 (15-oz.) cans garbanzo beans, rinsed and drained	1 lb. collard greens, thick stems removed and leaves chopped
1 rutabaga, peeled and cut into ¾-in. cubes	½ tsp. salt
½ large yellow onion, chopped	¼ tsp. freshly ground black pepper
3 tsp. garlic, minced	1½ cups uncooked brown rice
1 bay leaf	½ cup black olives, pitted and sliced
8 cups water	1 cup nonfat plain Greek-style yogurt
5 tsp. curry powder	
2 tsp. chili powder, or to taste	

1. Place garbanzo beans, rutabaga, onion, garlic, and bay leaf in a 5- to 7-quart slow cooker and add 5 cups water. Cover with lid and cook on high for 3 to 5 hours, or on low 8 to 10 hours.

2. About 30 to 45 minutes before the chickpea mixture is done cooking, stir in curry and chili powders. Add about half the greens and replace lid for 5 minutes, until wilted. Then add the remaining greens and continue cooking until chickpeas are tender. Stir in salt and black pepper. Remove bay leaf.

3. Meanwhile, combine rice and 3 cups water in a small saucepan and bring to a boil over high heat. Reduce heat to low, cover, and simmer for 50 minutes. Remove from heat.

4. Serve chickpeas over rice and top with black olives and yogurt.

HEALTHY NOTE

If your vegetarian style is to be dairy free, omit the yogurt in this recipe.

White Bean Chili with Quinoa

Italian spices and vegetables elevate the flavor of beans and quinoa.

Yield:	Prep time:	Cook time:	Serving size:
8 cups	10 minutes	26 minutes	1 cup

Each serving has:				
424 calories	1.9 g total fat	0 g saturated fat	0 mg cholesterol	36 mg sodium
77.3 g carbohydrates	19.3 g fiber	6.4 g sugars	27.9 g protein	

½ cup uncooked quinoa

4 cups water

1 large red bell pepper, cored, seeded, and chopped into ½-in. pieces

1 large green bell pepper, cored, seeded, and chopped into ½-in. pieces

1 tsp. ground chipotle pepper

2 (15-oz.) cans white beans, rinsed and drained

4 large fresh tomatoes, chopped with juices

1 tsp. dried oregano

1 tsp. dried thyme

4 cups fresh spinach, chopped

1. In a 4-quart saucepan, combine quinoa and water and place over high heat. Bring to a boil and then reduce heat to low. Cover and simmer for 15 minutes.

2. Add bell peppers, chipotle pepper, beans, tomatoes, oregano, and thyme to quinoa. Bring to a simmer and cook, uncovered, for about 10 minutes. When chili is thick, stir in spinach and cook for 1 more minute, until wilted. Serve hot.

TABLE TALK

Quinoa is a relatively new grain to American cuisine. It comes to us from South America and is closely related to beets and spinach.

Cannellini Beans with Greek Salad

Beans are added to a traditional Greek salad flavored with oregano, feta, and kalamata olives.

Yield:	Prep time:	Cook time:	Serving size:
10 cups	15 minutes	None	1²/₃ cups

Each serving has:			
348 calories	11.5 g total fat	3.1 g saturated fat	11 mg cholesterol 342 mg sodium
53.5 g carbohydrates	20.8 g fiber	7.3 g sugars	20.6 g protein

3 TB. olive oil

3 TB. red wine vinegar

2 TB. lemon juice

1 tsp. garlic, minced

¼ tsp. salt

½ tsp. pepper

4 cups mixed field greens

1 (15-oz.) can cannellini beans, rinsed and drained

5 plum tomatoes, cut lengthwise, cut into eighths

2 cucumbers, halved lengthwise, cut into chunks

3 TB. fresh oregano, minced

½ cup crumbled feta cheese

12 kalamata olives, pitted

1. In a large salad bowl, whisk together oil, vinegar, lemon juice, garlic, salt, and pepper.

2. Add greens, beans, tomatoes, cucumbers, and oregano to the salad bowl, and toss to mix.

3. Arrange salad on 6 plates and top each with feta and olives.

TABLE TALK

Find canned cannellini beans at the health-food store or specialty grocers.

Apple Baked Beans

Apple adds sweetness to baked beans that are served with a barley and broccoli salad.

Yield:	Prep time:	Cook time:	Serving size:
8 cups	15 minutes	50 minutes	1⅓ cups

Each serving has:				
419 calories	6.5 g total fat	0.9 g saturated fat	0 mg cholesterol	215 mg sodium
72.9 g carbohydrates	24.4 g fiber	7.2 g sugars	20.7 g protein	

2 TB. olive oil

½ medium yellow onion, chopped

1 (15-oz.) can navy beans, rinsed and drained

1 apple, cored and coarsely chopped

1 TB. brown mustard

¾ tsp. cinnamon

¾ tsp. ground dried ginger

1 TB. balsamic vinegar

½ tsp. salt

2 TB. water

2 cups cooked barley

½ cup radish, sliced

2 cups broccoli slaw

1½ tsp. red wine vinegar

1. Preheat oven to 325°F. Oil a 2-quart casserole dish with 1 teaspoon oil and set aside.

2. In a medium nonstick skillet, sauté onion in 2 teaspoons oil over medium heat for 5 minutes or until onion is translucent.

3. Combine beans with onions in the casserole dish. Stir in apple, mustard, cinnamon, ginger, balsamic vinegar, salt, and water. Cover with aluminum foil and bake for 45 minutes.

4. About 5 minutes before beans are done, in a medium bowl, place barley, radish, broccoli slaw, red wine vinegar, and remaining 1 tablespoon oil. Toss to combine. Serve baked beans alongside broccoli salad.

HEALTHY NOTE

This dish is high in fiber—from the beans, the slaw, and the apple.

Vegetarian Tacos

Each taco holds black beans flavored with cumin and chili powder, with a fresh vegetable topping.

Yield:	Prep time:	Cook time:	Serving size:
6 tacos	5 minutes	3 to 6 minutes	1 taco

Each serving has:				
441 calories	12.2 g total fat	2.9 g saturated fat	8 mg cholesterol	242 mg sodium
58.6 g carbohydrates	14.2 g fiber	3.4 g sugars	26.6 g protein	

6 hard corn taco shells

1 (15-oz.) can black beans, rinsed and drained

$\frac{1}{2}$ tsp. cumin

$\frac{1}{2}$ tsp. chili powder

2 medium tomatoes, diced

$\frac{1}{4}$ cup yellow or white onion, diced

1 cup iceberg lettuce, chopped

2 cups low-fat cheddar cheese, shredded

1 avocado, peeled, seeded, and cut into 6 wedges

1. Warm taco shells by microwaving on high for 15 seconds.

2. Place beans, cumin, and chili powder in a small saucepan over medium heat and warm for 3 to 5 minutes, stirring until heated throughout.

3. Fill each taco shell with beans, tomato, onion, lettuce, and cheese. Top with avocado wedge.

TABLE TALK

For an open-faced taco, use a soft flat corn tortilla and top with the ingredients. You can eat with a fork or roll up and eat as a soft taco.

Veggie Burgers

Yams, green peas, and carrots add natural sweetness to these garlic-flavored burgers.

Yield:	Prep time:	Cook time:	Serving size:
6 burgers	10 minutes	21 minutes	1 burger

Each serving has:				
195 calories	6.6 g total fat	1.3 g saturated fat	71 mg cholesterol	373 mg sodium
26.5 g carbohydrates	4.6 g fiber	6.3 g sugars	7.8 g protein	

1 TB. plus 1 tsp. olive oil	2 carrots, grated
2 green onions, minced	2 large eggs, beaten
1 tsp. garlic, minced	1 cup finely crumbled soft stone-ground breadcrumbs
2 cups frozen green peas, thawed	
1 medium yam, cooked until firm-tender, peeled, and grated	1 tsp. salt
	¼ tsp. paprika

1. In a small nonstick skillet, heat 1 teaspoon olive oil over medium heat. Add onions and garlic. Sauté until tender, about 5 minutes.

2. In a large bowl, mash peas lightly with a fork. Add green onion mixture, yam, carrots, eggs, ½ cup breadcrumbs, salt, and paprika to peas. Shape into 8 patties and then dredge in remaining ½ cup breadcrumbs.

3. In a large nonstick skillet, heat 2 tablespoons oil over medium heat. Add half the patties and cook, until lightly browned, about 4 minutes per side. Repeat with remaining patties.

TABLE TALK

Use day-old stone-ground bread for the breadcrumbs. Tear into small pieces and pulse in the food processor several times until you have uniformly sized crumbs.

Portobello Burgers

Portobello mushrooms add a robust flavor to these otherwise traditional burgers.

Yield:	Prep time:	Cook time:	Serving size:
4 burgers	20 minutes	12 minutes	1 burger

Each serving has:				
328 calories	7.5 g total fat	0.8 g saturated fat	2 mg cholesterol	479 mg sodium
51.4 g carbohydrates	6.7 g fiber	11.8 g sugars	18.4 g protein	

8 portobello mushrooms (3-oz. each), stems discarded	3-oz. low-fat cream cheese
1 TB. olive oil	4 slices sweet onion
4 stone-ground wheat rolls, sliced	1 tomato, cut in 4 slices
	8 red lettuce leaves

1. With a spoon, scrape black gills out of mushroom caps.

2. Brush oil on both sides of mushroom caps and let stand 20 minutes.

3. Preheat the broiler. Lightly oil a baking sheet.

4. Arrange mushrooms in one layer, gill side up, on the baking sheet. Broil 6 inches from the heat for 6 minutes or until somewhat soft. Turn and cook until mushrooms are hot and tender, about 6 minutes more.

5. Place a mushroom, gill side up, on a bottom bun. Spread with cream cheese. Add a second mushroom, gill side down, along with a tomato slice, an onion slice, two lettuce leaves, and the top bun.

HEALTHY NOTE

If you prefer to avoid dairy, substitute crumbled tofu for the cream cheese in this recipe. If you are gluten intolerant, use lettuce leaves as a wrap for your burger.

Curry with Portobello Mushrooms

Mushrooms and rice are flavored with coconut milk and ginger and topped with cashews.

Yield:	Prep time:	Cook time:	Serving size:
7 cups	10 minutes	21 to 26 minutes	1¾ cups

Each serving has:				
319 calories	15.4 g total fat	7.7 g saturated fat	0 mg cholesterol	313 mg sodium
40.1 g carbohydrates	3.6 g fiber	4.7 g sugars	8.8 g protein	

¾ cup basmati rice	1 TB. olive oil
1½ cups water	½ cup green onions, sliced
½ cup unsweetened coconut milk	2 tsp. curry powder
½ cup fresh cilantro, snipped	⅛ tsp. crushed red pepper
4 tsp. fresh ginger, finely minced	1 cup cherry tomatoes, halved or quartered
2 tsp. garlic, minced	½ tsp. salt
1 TB. lime juice	½ tsp. freshly ground black pepper
1 lb. portobello mushrooms, cut into ½-in. slices	4 TB. cashews, coarsely chopped

1. In a medium saucepan, combine rice and water, and bring to a boil. Reduce heat. Simmer, covered, 15 to 20 minutes or until rice is tender and water is absorbed.

2. Meanwhile, in a food processor, combine ¼ cup coconut milk, cilantro, 1 teaspoon ginger, 1 teaspoon garlic, and lime juice. Process until nearly smooth. Stir mixture into rice. Cover to keep warm.

3. In a large nonstick skillet, cook mushrooms in hot oil over medium heat for 5 minutes; turn occasionally. Add green onions, curry powder, red pepper, remaining 3 teaspoons ginger, and 1 teaspoon garlic. Cook and stir 1 minute. Stir in tomatoes and remaining ¼ cup coconut milk. Heat through. Season with salt and pepper.

4. To serve, divide rice among plates. Top with mushroom mixture and sprinkle with cashews.

Quinoa Stuffed Peppers

Green peppers are stuffed with a flavorful barley and quinoa mixture.

Yield:	Prep time:	Cook time:	Serving size:
4 peppers	25 minutes	45 minutes	1 pepper

Each serving has:				
252 calories	10.3 g total fat	2.4 g saturated fat	6 mg cholesterol	213 mg sodium
27.9 g carbohydrates	7.1 g fiber	7.6 g sugars	13.6 g protein	

1¾ cups water

¼ cup quick-cooking barley

¼ cup quinoa

2 TB. olive oil

2 tsp. garlic, minced

2 cups fresh white or crimini mushrooms, sliced

¼ tsp. freshly ground black pepper

1 (14.5 oz.) can low-sodium diced tomatoes, undrained

½ a 10-oz. package frozen chopped spinach, thawed and well drained

1 cup low-fat cheddar cheese, shredded

4 large green bell peppers

1. Preheat oven to 400°F. In a medium saucepan, bring water to boiling. Add barley and quinoa. Return to boiling. Reduce heat to high simmer. Cook, covered, for 12 minutes or until tender. Drain, reserving cooking liquid.

2. In a large nonstick skillet, heat oil over medium-high heat. Add garlic and mushrooms. Cook and stir 4 to 5 minutes or until mushrooms are tender. Stir in black pepper, tomatoes, and spinach. Stir in quinoa/barley mixture and ½ cup cheese. Remove from heat.

3. Remove pepper tops. Remove and discard seeds and membranes from peppers. Cut a small slice from the bottom of each pepper so that each stands up straight. Fill peppers with quinoa mixture. Place peppers, filled sides up, in a 2-quart square baking dish. Pour reserved cooking liquid into dish around peppers.

4. Bake, covered, for 35 minutes. Uncover and top each with remaining cheese. Bake, uncovered, for 10 minutes until peppers are tender and cheese is browned.

TABLE TALK

For a sweeter taste, use red or orange bell peppers in place of the green.

Side Dishes and Desserts

Our recipes make it easy to eat the recommended 5 to 10 servings of vegetables and fruit every day. The dishes in this part will wow your taste buds and make eating your vegetables a delicious event. Enjoy the varied seasonings as these recipes complement the main course, breakfast, and lunch offerings in this book.

Knowing how to fix whole grains will no longer be a mystery. Our cooking instructions are easy, and you'll find the grains filling. They add extra carbohydrate fuel to your body, to give you more endurance and stamina for an active lifestyle. Because grains are high in starch and too much starch can cause inflammation, be sure to eat only the recommended serving size so you don't overload on whole grains.

The legume recipes also take the mystery out of the hours-long process of preparing dry beans. And in a pinch, you can use already-cooked canned beans. Beans offer you protein and also high-energy starches. Eat the recommended amounts as you would the grains, and you'll enjoy lower inflammation levels.

Salads

Chapter 13

In This Chapter

- Anti-inflammatory salads
- An assorted rainbow of vegetables
- Light side salads to main-course entrées
- A variety of tasty dressings

The dressing *on* the salad is every bit as important as the vegetables and proteins *in* the salad. That's because the dressings contain anti-inflammatory properties, too.

Here's how it works: as few as 2 teaspoons of vinegar or lemon juice can lower the glycemic effect of a meal by one third. This helps keep your blood sugar in a healthy range and prevents insulin levels from spiking. Remember that elevated blood sugar and insulin levels increase a person's inflammation levels.

Our salad dressings contain vinegar or lemon juice, as well as healthy good oils, such as olive or walnut oil.

Don't make the mistake of avoiding salad dressings as a way to lose weight. The body can best absorb the vitamins and minerals in vegetables when they're eaten with a fat, preferably a healthy fat. The more nourished you are, the less likely you are to overeat or binge.

Enjoy these salads as interesting and delicious foods, but also know that you are winning in creating a healthier body as you eat.

Spinach Pomegranate Salad

Spinach and celery are tossed with a tangy combination of olive oil, capers, and green olives, and then topped with succulent orange, lemon, and pomegranate.

Yield:	Prep time:	Cook time:	Serving size:
6 cups	20 minutes	None	1½ cups

Each serving has:				
131 calories	7.6 g total fat	1.1 g saturated fat	0 mg cholesterol	212 mg sodium
15.5 g carbohydrates	4.4 g fiber	10.8 g sugars	2.2 g protein	

1 (10-oz.) package (8 cups) baby spinach, gently torn	2 TB. green olives, chopped
2 cups celery, finely diced	1 orange, peeled and sliced
2 TB. olive oil	1 lemon, peeled and sliced
1 TB. capers, drained	Seeds from 1 pomegranate

1. Place spinach and celery in a large bowl. Toss with olive oil, capers, and olives. Arrange on a serving dish.

2. Place orange and lemon slices on top of salad, and then sprinkle with pomegranate seeds. Serve at once.

TABLE TALK

To quickly remove seeds from the pomegranate, fill a large bowl with water. Score the pomegranate skin in wedges, being careful not to cut all the way into the seeds. Place the pomegranate in the water, and carefully pull apart the segments and loosen the seeds from the pulp. The seeds will fall to the bottom of the bowl, and the pulp will float. When you have loosened all the seeds, remove the pulp and drain the water from the seeds.

Pink Grapefruit Salad with Walnuts

Walnuts grace a salad of spinach and tangy grapefruit, dressed with fragrant olive oil.

Yield:	Prep time:	Cook time:	Serving size:
8 cups	15 minutes	None	1⅓ cups

Each serving has:				
185 calories	16.2 g total fat	1.5 g saturated fat	1 mg cholesterol	88 mg sodium
7.6 g carbohydrates	2.6 g fiber	4 g sugars	5.4 g protein	

3 TB. olive oil

Juice of 1 orange, about ¼ cup

1 tsp. orange zest

⅛ tsp. salt

⅛ tsp. freshly ground black pepper

10 oz. (8 cups) spinach leaves, gently torn

¾ cup walnuts, coarsely chopped

2 medium pink grapefruits, peeled and divided into segments

1. In a medium jar with a lid, place olive oil, orange juice, orange zest, salt, and pepper. Shake to blend.

2. Place spinach in a large salad bowl and toss with orange juice dressing.

3. Arrange salad on 4 plates. Top with equally divided walnuts and grapefruit segments.

TABLE TALK

To remove the skin from each grapefruit segment, first peel the grapefruit. Use a paring knife to slit the membrane, and then peel it away with your fingers. For a quicker solution, purchase 2 (15-ounce) cans unsweetened pink grapefruit segments and drain before using.

Salmon Salad Niçoise

Dijon mustard, anchovies, and garlic add a French flavor flair to this hearty salad.

Yield:	Prep time:	Cook time:	Serving size:
10 cups	20 minutes	10 minutes	1²/₃ cups

Each serving has:

292 calories	11.7 g total fat	2.5 g saturated fat	154 mg cholesterol	144 mg sodium
29.8 g carbohydrates	4.8 g fiber	3.6 g sugars	18.6 g protein	

½ lb. fresh green beans, rinsed, with ends trimmed

2 yams, cut into 1-in. pieces

1 TB. red wine vinegar

1 tsp. Dijon mustard

1 tsp. 100% anchovy paste

1 tsp. garlic, minced

1 TB. olive oil

1 lb. romaine lettuce, rinsed, dried, trimmed, and torn into bite-size pieces

4 eggs, hard boiled, peeled, and sliced

10 oz. salmon, canned or pouched in water

1. Fill a medium pot one-third full with water and boil over high heat. When water comes to a boil, add beans and yams. Reduce heat to medium and simmer for 5 minutes or until the tip of a knife easily pierces yams. Drain and set aside to cool. Chop beans into 1-inch lengths.

2. Place vinegar, mustard, anchovy paste, garlic, and olive oil in a screw-top lidded medium or small jar. Shake ingredients until blended.

3. Place romaine in large salad bowl. Toss with dressing.

4. Divide romaine onto 6 serving plates. Top each with equal amounts of beans, yams, egg slices, and salmon. Serve at once.

TABLE TALK

The classic salad niçoise calls for tuna and anchovy fillets. You can substitute anchovy fillets for the anchovy paste in this recipe or omit them if you prefer a milder taste.

Pear and Jicama Slaw

Enjoy the flavors of poppy seeds and green onions in this unique slaw.

Yield:	Prep time:	Cook time:	Serving size:
8 cups	30 minutes	None	1⅓ cups

Each serving has:				
145 calories	3.7 g total fat	0.6 g saturated fat	3 g cholesterol	261 g sodium
28.6 g carbohydrates	5.5 g fiber	13.5 g sugars	2 g protein	

¼ cup low-fat mayonnaise

2 TB. red wine vinegar

1 tsp. poppy seeds

¼ tsp. salt

¼ tsp. freshly ground black pepper

2 pears, cut into matchsticks

1 small jicama, peeled and cut into matchsticks

2 medium carrots, cut into matchsticks

¼ cup green onions, chopped

1. Whisk mayonnaise, vinegar, poppy seeds, salt, and pepper in a large bowl. Add pears, jicama, carrots, and onion, and toss to coat. Serve immediately.

TABLE TALK

Poppy seeds add visual sparkle and a sweet taste to this salad.

Orange Couscous Salad with Dates

Eating this salad will transport you to a desert oasis due to its combined flavors of mint, cilantro, dates, and couscous.

Yield:	Prep time:	Cook time:	Serving size:
16 cups	40 minutes	None	2 cups

Each serving has:				
370 calories	16.6 g total fat	1.4 g saturated fat	0 mg cholesterol	29 mg sodium
48.4 g carbohydrates	7.1 g fiber	14.8 g sugars	11.1 g protein	

1½ cups couscous

1½ cups boiling water

10 dates, seeded and coarsely chopped

1 cup toasted walnuts, chopped coarsely

¼ cup orange juice

3 TB. walnut oil

3 TB. olive oil

2 TB. cider vinegar

½ tsp. ground coriander

1 large grapefruit, peeled and sliced thinly

2 medium oranges, peeled and sliced thinly

14 trimmed red radishes, sliced thinly

3 cups mixed salad greens

2 cups loosely packed fresh mint leaves

2 cups loosely packed fresh cilantro

1. Combine couscous with water in a large heatproof bowl. Cover and let stand about 5 minutes or until water is absorbed, fluffing with fork occasionally. Cool 10 minutes; stir in dates and walnuts.

2. In a small bowl, whisk together orange juice, walnut oil, olive oil, vinegar, and coriander to make dressing.

3. Add grapefruit, oranges, radishes, salad greens, mint, and cilantro to couscous mixture. Pour dressing over salad and toss. Serve immediately or refrigerate up to 4 days until ready to serve.

HEALTHY NOTE

Eating a wide variety of green vegetables and herbs, such as the mint and cilantro in this recipe, gives you added benefits for fighting inflammation.

Chicken Antipasto Salad

Roasting the eggplant, and zucchini in this recipe intensifies their tastes and makes them softer. The vinaigrette dressing sets off their unique flavors.

Yield:	Prep time:	Cook time:	Serving size:
20 cups	30 minutes	20 minutes	2½ cups

Each serving has:

237 calories	12.8 g total fat	2.6 g saturated fat	97 mg cholesterol	300 mg sodium
20.2 g carbohydrates	8.9 g fiber	7 g sugars	22.5 g protein	

2 large eggs, hard boiled and quartered	1 (15-oz.) jar roasted red bell peppers, drained and thinly sliced
1½ TB. drained capers	1 (12-oz.) jar marinated quartered artichokes, drained
3 TB. white wine vinegar	
3 TB. fresh oregano, coarsely chopped	1 lb. cooked chicken breasts, sliced thinly
1 tsp. garlic, minced	14 oz. (9 cups) mixed salad greens, trimmed
4 TB. olive oil	
4 baby eggplants, sliced thinly	
2 large zucchini, sliced thinly	

1. Preheat oven to 450°F.

2. In a food processor, process eggs, capers, vinegar, oregano, and garlic until finely chopped. With motor running, add 3 tablespoons olive oil in a thin, steady stream until dressing thickens.

3. Place eggplants and zucchini on two rimmed baking sheets. Brush with 1 tablespoon olive oil. Bake for 15 to 18 minutes until just tender. Cool.

4. Place bell peppers, eggplants, and zucchini in a large bowl with artichokes, chicken, and egg-caper dressing; toss gently to combine. Serve over mixed salad greens.

HEALTHY NOTE

This salad gives you almost four servings of vegetables and plenty of antioxidants to keep your diet anti-inflammatory and delicious.

Turkey Salad with Beans and Peas

Lemon juice and mustard dress this high-fiber and high-protein salad and add succulent flavor.

Yield:	Prep time:	Cook time:	Serving size:
12 cups	20 minutes	None	1½ cups

Each serving has:				
327 calories	8.3 g total fat	0.9 g saturated fat	45 mg cholesterol	540 mg sodium
33.4 g carbohydrates	12.8 g fiber	5.5 g sugars	32.3 g protein	

2 TB. lemon juice	¼ cup fresh mint, coarsely chopped
1 TB. whole-grain mustard	1 cup mung bean sprouts
2 TB. white wine vinegar	2 cups baby arugula
3 TB. olive oil	1½ lb. low-sodium turkey breast, sliced
2 cups fresh fava beans, shelled	
1¾ cups frozen green peas	
2 cups sugar snap peas, trimmed	

1. Whisk together lemon juice, mustard, vinegar, and olive oil.

2. Place fava beans in a steamer basket set in a saucepan with water. Cover the pan and boil water. Cook beans until just tender. Drain and then rinse under cold water. Drain again. Peel away gray-colored outer shells.

3. Meanwhile, steam green peas and sugar snap peas until just tender; drain. Rinse under cold water and drain again.

4. Place beans and pea mixture in a large bowl with mint, sprouts, arugula, and lemon-mustard dressing. Toss gently to combine. Place slices of turkey on top of salad.

HEALTHY NOTE

The legumes (fava beans) and peas in this recipe make it very high in fiber and protein.

Pastrami, Beet, and Yam Salad

Horseradish and lemon add tang and heat to this salad filled with hearty vegetables.

Yield:	Prep time:	Cook time:	Serving size:
8 cups	30 minutes	10 minutes	2 cups

Each serving has:				
321 calories	12.2 g total fat	2.6 g saturated fat	67 mg cholesterol	502 mg sodium
39.4 g carbohydrates	6.7 g fiber	6 g sugars	13.9 g protein	

2 medium yams, cut into 1½-in. pieces

1 TB. prepared horseradish

1½ TB. lemon juice

¼ cup olive oil

1½ tsp. red wine vinegar

7 red radishes, trimmed and thinly sliced

4 cups red leaf lettuce, trimmed

1½ cups all-natural lean pastrami, torn into bite-size pieces

2 cups cucumber, sliced

3 TB. fresh dill, coarsely chopped

3 medium fresh beets, peeled and coarsely grated

1. Place yams in a large saucepan and add enough water to cover them. Boil yams until just tender. Drain. Cool for 10 minutes.

2. Meanwhile, stir together horseradish, lemon juice, olive oil, and vinegar.

3. Combine yams and radishes in a large bowl with lettuce, pastrami, cucumber, and dill.

4. Divide pastrami salad among 6 serving plates. Top with beets and drizzle with horseradish dressing.

HEALTHY NOTE

This anti-inflammation salad is a great way to enjoy the taste of pastrami without eating ingredients that cause inflammation: too much salt, wheat, or high-cholesterol cheese.

Pork and Coconut Salad

A spicy Thai dressing adds Asian flavor to lean pork and fresh vegetables.

Yield:	Prep time:	Cook time:	Serving size:
10 cups	40 minutes	10 minutes	$1\frac{1}{3}$ cups

Each serving has:			
308 calories	14.4 g total fat	8.6 g saturated fat	83 mg cholesterol 555 mg sodium
11.6 g carbohydrates	2.8 g fiber	4 g sugars	34.2 g protein

3 TB. lime juice

$1\frac{1}{2}$ TB. fish sauce

$1\frac{1}{2}$ TB. sweet Thai chili sauce

$\frac{3}{4}$ cup unsweetened coconut milk

$1\frac{1}{2}$ lb. pork fillets, trimmed

1 TB. olive oil

3 TB. lime juice

$1\frac{1}{4}$ lb. bok choy, quartered

2 large carrots, cut into matchsticks

$\frac{1}{2}$ cup fresh basil, coarsely chopped

$\frac{1}{2}$ cup fresh cilantro, coarsely chopped

$1\frac{1}{4}$ cups bean sprouts

4 green onions, sliced thinly

2 TB. shredded unsweetened coconut

1. In a small bowl, whisk together lime juice, fish sauce, chili sauce, and coconut milk to make dressing.

2. Toss together pork, oil, and lime juice in a medium bowl.

3. Cook pork on heated grill or grill pan until browned and juices run clear. Let stand for 5 minutes. Slice pork thinly.

4. Meanwhile, steam bok choy until just wilted, about 3 minutes.

5. Place pork, bok choy, carrots, basil, cilantro, bean sprouts, onions, and shredded coconut in a large bowl with dressing. Toss gently to combine. Serve immediately.

HEALTHY NOTE

Coconut is technically high in saturated fat, but it also contains healthful conjugated linoleic acids, which aid with weight loss and soothe inflammation.

Smoked Salmon with Fruit Salad

The sweetness of the cantaloupe, fennel, and grapes is balanced with the tangy flavor of the yogurt dressing in this recipe.

Yield:	Prep time:		Cook time:		Serving size:
14 cups	15 minutes		None		1¾ cups

Each serving has:				
100 calories	4.6 g total fat	0.8 g saturated fat	6 mg cholesterol	457 mg sodium
9.7 g carbohydrates	1.9 g fiber	6.9 g sugars	5.8 g protein	

½ (6-oz.) carton plain low-fat yogurt

2 TB. olive oil

2 TB. lemon juice

1 tsp. garlic, minced

½ tsp. ground cardamom

½ tsp. freshly ground black pepper

8 cups romaine lettuce, torn in bite-size pieces

2 cups cantaloupe, cut into thin wedges

2 cups fennel, thinly sliced

1 cup red grapes

6 oz. smoked salmon, broken into bite-size pieces

1. In a small bowl, whisk together yogurt, olive oil, lemon juice, garlic, cardamom, and pepper.

2. On a serving platter, arrange romaine. Top with cantaloupe, fennel, grapes, and salmon.

3. Drizzle dressing on salad. Serve immediately.

TABLE TALK

Be sure to purchase plain yogurt that contains beneficial probiotics and states this on the label.

Ham with Black and White Bean Salad

Oregano and paprika add bright flavor to the beans and ham in this dish.

Yield:	Prep time:	Cook time:	Serving size:
8 cups	10 minutes	None	$\frac{4}{5}$ cup

Each serving has:				
410 calories	7.9 g total fat	1.7 g saturated fat	15 mg cholesterol	400 mg sodium
62.8 g carbohydrates	14.7 g fiber	3.7 g sugars	25.2 g protein	

1 (15-oz.) can white beans, rinsed and drained

1 (15-oz.) can black beans, rinsed and drained

1 (16-oz.) package frozen whole-kernel corn, thawed and drained

1 medium red onion, chopped

2 cups ham, cubed (about ½ lb.)

3 TB. red wine vinegar

3 TB. olive oil

½ tsp. paprika

1 tsp. oregano

¼ tsp. freshly ground black pepper

1. Place white and black beans in a large salad bowl. Add corn, onion, and ham. Mix well.

2. In a small bowl, whisk together vinegar, olive oil, paprika, oregano, and pepper. Pour over bean mixture and toss. Refrigerate until ready to serve.

HEALTHY NOTE

This salad delivers lots of fiber and protein in a concentrated healthful recipe. Because of this, a small portion can go a long way toward satisfying your hunger. This is a superb salad for packed lunches and late-afternoon snacks.

Tuna Salad with Apples

Apples and red bell pepper add crunch and brightness to the tuna, while the Dijon mustard and tarragon dressing complete the flavor combination.

Yield:	Prep time:	Cook time:	Serving size:
9 cups	10 minutes	None	1½ cups

Each serving has:				
194 calories	11.3 g total fat	1.5 g saturated fat	15 mg cholesterol	123 mg sodium
13.5 g carbohydrates	3.9 g fiber	7.2 g sugars	9.8 g protein	

3 TB. olive oil

3 TB. cider vinegar

1 tsp. Dijon mustard

½ tsp. dried tarragon

¼ cup low-fat mayonnaise

1 (6-oz.) can tuna in water, drained

1 apple, cored and chopped

1 (10-oz.) package frozen green peas, thawed and drained

1 red bell pepper, cored, seeded, and chopped

3 cups iceberg lettuce, shredded

1. Whisk together olive oil, vinegar, mustard, tarragon, and mayonnaise in a small bowl, and set aside.

2. In a large bowl, combine tuna, apple, peas, and bell pepper. Pour dressing mixture over salad and toss to blend.

3. Serve over bed of shredded lettuce.

TABLE TALK

Prepare this quick salad when you have limited time yet want a superb meal high in nutrition. You can store it in the refrigerator for up to four days.

Crab Salad with Watermelon and Avocado

This unique combination of ingredients gives you the best of summer in one salad. Crab, watermelon, and avocado share top billing with the added flavors of cilantro and black pepper.

Yield:	Prep time:	Cook time:	Serving size:
8 cups	10 minutes	None	1⅓ cups

Each serving has:				
223 calories	11.3 g total fat	0.6 g saturated fat	76 mg cholesterol	315 mg sodium
15.3 g carbohydrates	5.3 g fiber	7.6 g sugars	17.5 g protein	

1 lb. crab, cooked and shelled	2 avocados, peeled, pitted, and chopped
4 cups seedless watermelon, chopped	¼ tsp. salt
1 medium red onion, sliced	¼ tsp. freshly ground black pepper
½ cup fresh cilantro, chopped	6 large Bibb lettuce leaves

1. In a large salad bowl, combine crab, watermelon, onion, cilantro, avocados, salt, and pepper.

2. Place 1 lettuce leaf on each of 6 serving plates and top with salad.

TABLE TALK

Purchase crab meat in cans or pouches to save time when making this recipe.

Artichoke Molded Salad

This savory aspic is flavored with Italian herbs and garlic for a wonderful side dish.

Yield:	Prep time:	Cook time:	Serving size:
8 cups	15 minutes	None	1 cup

Each serving has:				
210 calories	13.6 g total fat	2.9 g saturated fat	21 mg cholesterol	495 mg sodium
12.2 g carbohydrates	4.1 g fiber	0.1 g sugars	12 g protein	

1 (1-oz.) packet unflavored gelatin	5 green onions with tops, finely chopped
¾ cup water	1½ cups low-fat mozzarella cheese, shredded
1 cup low-fat mayonnaise	
1 (14-oz.) can artichoke hearts, drained and chopped	1 tsp. Italian herb seasoning
½ (10-oz.) package frozen green peas, thawed	½ tsp. garlic powder
	¼ tsp. salt
2 TB. lemon juice	8 large Bibb lettuce leaves
1 (4-oz.) jar pimentos, chopped	

1. Soften gelatin in ¼ cup cold water in a large bowl. Boil remaining ½ cup water and mix into gelatin. Add mayonnaise and stir until smooth.

2. Stir artichoke hearts, peas, lemon juice, pimentos, onions, cheese, Italian herb seasoning, garlic powder, and salt into gelatin mixture.

3. Pour gelatin mixture into a ring mold and refrigerate for at least 2 hours, or until set.

4. Slip a knife around edges to loosen from the mold. Unmold onto a serving plate lined with lettuce.

TABLE TALK

When preparing any recipe with gelatin in the hot summer months, add a teaspoon of white vinegar to the mix. It will help keep your salads and desserts firm.

Lobster and Orange Salad

Lobster is deliciously paired with oranges and shallots, while balsamic vinegar and thyme lend additional flavor.

Yield:	Prep time:	Cook time:	Serving size:
14 cups	30 minutes	8 to 12 minutes	1¾ cups

Each serving has:				
194 calories	6.2 g total fat	1 g saturated fat	165 mg cholesterol	563 mg sodium
11.2 g carbohydrates	2.6 g fiber	8.1 g sugars	22.9 g protein	

6 cups water

4 (8-oz.) frozen lobster tails, thawed in the refrigerator

10 cups mesclun greens or other salad greens

3 medium oranges, peeled and sectioned

2 shallots, finely chopped

3 TB. olive oil

¼ cup balsamic vinegar

2 tsp. snipped fresh thyme or ¼ tsp. dried thyme, crushed

¼ tsp. freshly ground black pepper

1. In a 3-quart saucepan, bring water to boiling. Add lobster. Simmer, uncovered, for 8 to 12 minutes or until shells turn bright red and meat is tender. Drain; let stand until cool enough to handle.

2. In a large bowl, toss together greens and orange sections. Divide salad mixture among 4 dinner plates.

3. For dressing, in a medium skillet, cook shallots in hot oil until tender. Carefully add balsamic vinegar and thyme. Bring to boiling, and then reduce heat to just keep dressing warm.

4. To remove lobster meat from shell, insert a fork and push tail meat out in one piece. Remove and discard black vein that runs the length of tail meat. Slice tail meat, making ½-inch medallions.

5. Arrange lobster medallions on top of greens. Spoon warm dressing over salads and sprinkle with pepper. Serve immediately.

Variation: Substitute other types of shellfish for the lobster, such as crab, scallops, or shrimp.

TABLE TALK

This recipe calls for the salad to be served warm, but it's just as delicious chilled.

Sesame Asparagus Salad

An Asian-flavored dressing with rice vinegar, soy sauce, and ginger adds flavor to the spring vegetables.

Yield:	Prep time:	Cook time:	Serving size:
13 cups	25 minutes	2 to 4 minutes	1⅔ cups

Each serving has:				
129 calories	7.7 g total fat	1.1 g saturated fat	0 mg cholesterol	165 mg sodium
9.7 g carbohydrates	3.9 g fiber	5.1 g sugars	4.5 g protein	

1 lb. fresh asparagus, trimmed	⅛ tsp. freshly ground black pepper
1 lb. fresh snow peapods, trimmed	6 cups watercress, torn into bite-size pieces
½ cup rice vinegar	
¼ cup olive oil	2 medium yellow bell peppers, cored, seeded, and cut into strips
1 tsp. garlic, minced	
2 tsp. soy sauce	1 cup grape tomatoes
¾ tsp. ground ginger	1 TB. sesame seeds, toasted
¼ tsp. salt	

1. In a large saucepan, cook asparagus spears and peapods covered in a small amount of boiling water for 2 to 4 minutes or until crisp-tender. Drain. Rinse with cold water and then drain well again.

2. In a screw-top jar, combine rice vinegar, olive oil, garlic, soy sauce, ginger, salt, and pepper. Shake well.

3. In a very large bowl, toss together asparagus spears, peapods, watercress, bell peppers, and tomatoes. Add dressing and toss well. Sprinkle with sesame seeds.

TABLE TALK

To stop the cooking action, drain the vegetables and then rinse with cold water immediately. Then drain again before adding to the recipe.

Black-Eyed Pea Salad

A warm dressing gently wilts the salad greens and pops the flavor of the black-eyed peas in this dish.

Yield:	Prep time:	Cook time:	Serving size:
12 cups	15 minutes	None	2 cups

Each serving has:				
109 calories	3 g total fat	0 g saturated fat	0 mg cholesterol	42 mg sodium
16.8 g carbohydrates	4.8 g fiber	3.8 g sugars	5 g protein	

1 large sweet onion, chopped (1 cup)	2 cups radishes, washed, trimmed, and cut into large pieces
1 TB. olive oil	1 (15-oz.) can black-eyed peas, rinsed and drained
½ cup cider vinegar	8 green onions, trimmed
⅛ tsp. freshly ground black pepper	
8 cups mixed salad greens	

1. In a medium-to-large covered skillet, cook onion in olive oil over medium-low heat for 13 to 15 minutes or until onions are tender, stirring occasionally. Remove from stove. Stir in vinegar and pepper.

2. Place salad greens in a large salad bowl. Add radishes and black-eyed peas. Toss with vinaigrette. Top with green onions and serve.

HEALTHY NOTE

Be sure to use canned *organic* black-eyed peas in this recipe to further reduce the possibility of inflammation-causing components.

Red Cabbage with Apple Slaw

The dried cranberries and apple in this recipe add a sweet flavor that is balanced by the vinaigrette dressing.

Yield:	Prep time:	Cook time:	Serving size:
8 cups	20 minutes	None	1⅓ cups

Each serving has:

136 calories	9.3 g total fat	1.3 g saturated fat	3 mg cholesterol	150 mg sodium
13.6 g carbohydrates	3.4 g fiber	8.9 g sugars	1.1 g protein	

4 cups red cabbage, cut into 1-in. pieces

2 medium Golden Delicious apples, cored and cubed

2 medium carrots, sliced

2 TB. unsweetened dried cranberries

¼ cup olive oil

¼ cup red wine vinegar

1 TB. Dijon-style mustard

¼ tsp. salt

¼ tsp. freshly ground black pepper

1. In a large bowl, combine cabbage, apples, carrots, and cranberries.

2. In a small bowl, whisk together olive oil, vinegar, mustard, salt, and pepper. Add to salad and toss to coat. Serve at once or refrigerate, covered, for 2 to 24 hours.

TABLE TALK

If your local grocery store doesn't stock unsweetened dried cranberries, look for them at a health-food grocer.

Spinach Salad with Berries and Cheese

Blueberries and kiwi perk up the flavors of the spinach salad ingredients, including pistachios and blue cheese.

Yield:	Prep time:	Cook time:	Serving size:
10 cups	20 minutes	None	1⅔ cups

Each serving has:				
181 calories	13.5 g total fat	2.6 g saturated fat	4 mg cholesterol	102 mg sodium
12.6 g carbohydrates	3.1 g fiber	6.7 g sugars	4.8 g protein	

1¼ cups fresh or frozen blueberries

1 (6-oz.) package fresh baby spinach (about 8 cups)

2 kiwi, peeled and chopped

½ cup unsalted shelled pistachio nuts, chopped or whole

¼ cup low-fat blue cheese, crumbled (1 oz.)

¼ cup raspberry vinegar

3 TB. olive oil

1. Thaw berries, if frozen. In a large salad bowl, toss together 1 cup blueberries, spinach, kiwi, pistachios, and blue cheese.

2. In a food processor, combine ¼ cup blueberries, vinegar, and olive oil. Cover and process until smooth.

3. Pour dressing over salad mixture. Toss lightly to coat. Pass remaining dressing with salad.

Variation: Use strawberries or raspberries in place of the blueberries.

 HEALTHY NOTE

Nuts, as in this salad, add an enticing crunch and healthy nutritional oils and protein.

Plum and Walnut Salad

Ham and blue cheese offer a counterpoint to the sweet flavor of the plums in this dish.

Yield:	Prep time:	Cook time:	Serving size:
12 cups	20 minutes	None	1½ cups

Each serving has:			
127 calories	10.3 g total fat	1.9 g saturated fat	7 mg cholesterol 262 mg sodium
6.6 g carbohydrates	1.8 g fiber	3.8 g sugars	3.7 g protein

4 cups radicchio, torn in bite-size pieces	2 TB. white wine vinegar
4 cups baby spinach	2 TB. olive oil
4 plums, quartered and pitted	1 TB. Dijon-style mustard
½ cup walnuts, coarsely chopped and toasted	¼ tsp. salt
2 slices ham, cut into ½-in. strips	¼ tsp. freshly ground black pepper
	¼ cup blue cheese, crumbled

1. Place radicchio in a salad bowl with spinach, plums, walnuts, and ham.

2. In a small bowl, whisk together vinegar, olive oil, mustard, salt, and pepper. Drizzle on salad and toss gently to combine. Sprinkle with cheese and serve at once.

HEALTHY NOTE

Walnuts add an extra boost to your anti-inflammatory diet. They give you omega-3 essential fatty acids that help protect your heart and maintain a positive mental attitude.

Red Vegetable Slaw

Nutritious and healthy red vegetables add color, while the dressing adds a tangy and spicy flavor.

Yield:	Prep time:	Cook time:	Serving size:
10 cups	25 minutes	None	1 cup

Each serving has:				
102 calories	6.3 g total fat	2 g saturated fat	14 mg cholesterol	253 mg sodium
8.8 g carbohydrates	2.2 g fiber	5.5 g sugars	3 g protein	

⅓ cup low-fat sour cream

⅓ cup low-fat mayonnaise

1 tsp. paprika

¼ tsp. cayenne pepper

1 tsp. lemon juice

4 cups red cabbage, shredded

1 11½ oz. can sliced beets, drained

1 large red bell pepper, cut into thin strips

¾ cup radishes, trimmed and thinly sliced

1 large carrot, thinly sliced

4 oz. salami, thinly sliced and quartered

1. In a small bowl, whisk together sour cream, mayonnaise, paprika, cayenne pepper, and lemon juice.

2. In a large bowl, combine cabbage, beets, red pepper, radishes, carrot, and salami. Add dressing and toss to coat. Serve at once.

HEALTHY NOTE

The color of this salad indicates that it's filled with an abundance of powerful antioxidants.

Broccoli Salad with Lemon and Garlic

A tangy dressing fragrant with rosemary and lemon dresses up the healthy cruciferous vegetables of broccoli and cauliflower.

Yield:	Prep time:	Cook time:	Serving size:
8 cups	20 minutes	None	1 cup

Each serving has:				
119 calories	9.3 g total fat	1.3 g saturated fat	0 mg cholesterol	103 mg sodium
7.7 g carbohydrates	2.8 g fiber	2.9 g sugars	2.8 g protein	

⅓ cup red wine vinegar	1 (16-oz.) package broccoli slaw
⅓ cup olive oil	2 cups small cauliflower florets
2 tsp. garlic, minced	1 green bell pepper, cored, seeded, and chopped
1 tsp. fresh rosemary, snipped	1 large tomato, chopped
1 tsp. lemon zest, finely shredded	¼ cup fresh cilantro, snipped
2 TB. lemon juice	¼ cup fresh basil, snipped
¼ tsp. salt	
¼ tsp. freshly ground black pepper	

1. In a large screw-top jar, combine vinegar, olive oil, garlic, rosemary, lemon zest, lemon juice, salt, and pepper. Shake to blend.

2. In a large bowl, toss together broccoli slaw, cauliflower, bell pepper, tomato, cilantro, and basil.

3. Add dressing to the vegetable mixture, and toss to coat. Serve immediately, or cover and chill for up to 4 hours. Stir before serving.

TABLE TALK

This salad contains two cruciferous vegetables: broccoli and cauliflower. They're both high in vitamin C and soluble fiber and contain phytonutrients.

Fruit

In This Chapter

- Recipes that help you get your two servings of fruit daily
- Spices and herbs that add taste enhancement to fruit
- Unexpected fruit combinations
- Fruit chutneys and relishes to perk up entrées

Fruit can make you healthy. The time-tested adage "An apple a day keeps the doctor away" can also help you keep inflammation at bay.

Fruit's nutritional advantages are many:

- It offers plenty of soluble fiber and is easy to digest.

- Its natural sweetness satisfies your sweet tooth and sweet taste buds.

- It tastes delicious when served chilled and often when served warm.

- It's not just for summertime, but is widely available all year long.

- Eating organic fruit further lowers inflammation, as you avoid eating residual pesticides and fertilizers.

Purchase only the amount of fruit you can reasonably eat within a week. If stored much longer, it can become mealy and lose its crispness. Exceptions include apples, oranges, and grapefruit, which can hold in the refrigerator for several weeks, if you're lucky.

Pears Baked with Cream Cheese

Honey mustard flavors pears that are topped with walnuts.

Yield:	Prep time:	Cook time:	Serving size:
4 pear halves	10 minutes	35 minutes	1 pear half

Each serving has:				
157 calories	6.8 g total fat	1.7 g saturated fat	6 mg cholesterol	200 mg sodium
18.5 g carbohydrates	3.4 g fiber	11 g sugars	4 g protein	

1 TB. honey mustard

1 TB. olive oil

1 tsp. lemon juice

½ tsp. freshly ground black pepper

2 medium ripe pears, preferably Bosc

2 oz. reduced-fat cream cheese, cut into 4 slices

4 tsp. walnuts, chopped and toasted

1. Preheat oven to 425°F. Coat an 8-inch-square metal baking pan with cooking spray.

2. Whisk mustard, olive oil, lemon juice, and pepper in a small bowl.

3. Cut pears in half lengthwise, hollow out cores, and slice a small piece off the skin sides so they will lie flat when served. Brush all over with the mustard glaze and place cored side down in the prepared pan.

4. Bake pears for 30 minutes, basting half-way through with glaze. Gently turn them over, baste again, and place ¼ of cheese in the hollow of each pear. Bake until pears are tender and cheese is slightly softened, 3 to 5 minutes. Sprinkle each pear half with 1 teaspoon walnuts.

HEALTHY NOTE

This recipe offers you high-quality protein in the cheese and omega-3's from the walnuts while you enjoy the succulent baked pears.

Tangerine Watercress Salad

Chilies add heat and spice to this unique fruit-and-vegetable salad.

Yield:	Prep time:	Cook time:	Serving size:
9 cups	25 minutes	5 minutes	1½ cups

Each serving has:				
187 calories	8.8 g total fat	1 g saturated fat	0 mg cholesterol	30 mg sodium
25.7 g carbohydrates	4 g fiber	19.4 g sugars	5.3 g protein	

2 fresh small red Serrano or Thai chilies, chopped coarsely	1 cup frozen peas
2 tsp. garlic, minced	6 cups watercress, trimmed
2 TB. olive oil	½ cup toasted blanched almonds, slivered
3 TB. lemon juice	7 oz. seedless red grapes, halved lengthwise
4 medium tangerines (about 1¾ lb.), peeled	

1. Blend or process chilies, garlic, olive oil, and 1½ tablespoons lemon juice until smooth.

2. Supreme tangerines over a large bowl, to save juice. To do this, cut away the membrane from each segment. Reserve segments with juice.

3. Meanwhile, steam peas until just tender, about 5 minutes.

4. Place peas in the large bowl with tangerine segments and juice, watercress, almonds, grapes, chili mixture, and 1½ tablespoons remaining lemon juice; toss gently to combine. Serve immediately.

TABLE TALK

Don't be afraid of watercress—it's an excellent and somewhat exotic choice for salad greens. It's a leaf vegetable that's prized for its peppery and tangy flavor.

Waldorf Salad

Chicken, apples, celery, cucumber, and walnuts are wrapped in creamy yogurt in this delicious recipe.

Yield:	Prep time:	Cook time:	Serving size:
10 cups	15 minutes	None	1¼ cups

Each serving has:				
233 calories	11.8 g total fat	1.4 g saturated fat	54 mg cholesterol	211 mg sodium
11.2 g carbohydrates	2.2 g fiber	7.2 g sugars	20.9 g protein	

1 lb. cooked chicken breast, cubed	½ cup walnuts, coarsely chopped
2 apples, cored and chopped	1 (6-oz.) carton plain nonfat yogurt
1 cup (about 2 ribs) celery, chopped	½ cup low-fat mayonnaise
1 cup cucumber, chopped	5 cups shredded lettuce

1. Place chicken, apples, celery, cucumber, and walnuts in a large mixing bowl.

2. Stir together yogurt and mayonnaise in a small bowl. Add to salad and toss to mix well. May be served at room temperature or refrigerated for several hours. Serve over shredded lettuce.

HEALTHY NOTE

This low-fat version of a Waldorf salad dresses the crunchy fruit and vegetables with healthy yogurt. If you prefer to eat dairy free, omit the yogurt and add an extra ½ cup of low-fat mayonnaise.

Strawberries and Melon

Strawberries and cantaloupe are splashed with flavored balsamic vinegar and a pinch of salt, both of which highlight the sweet taste of the fruit.

Yield:	Prep time:	Cook time:	Serving size:
4 cups	15 minutes plus 15 to 45 minutes chill time	None	⅔ cup

Each serving has:

39 calories	0.3 g total fat	0 g saturated fat	0 mg cholesterol	2.8 mg sodium
9.3 g carbohydrates	2.1 g fiber	6.5 g sugars	0.8 g protein	

1 quart (1 lb.) strawberries, rinsed, hulled, and quartered	1 small cantaloupe, seeded, rind removed, and cut into 8 to 12 wedges
1 TB. flavored balsamic vinegar, your choice of flavor	Salt

1. Put strawberries and vinegar in a medium bowl, and toss gently to combine. Refrigerate, tossing occasionally, until just softened and juicy, for 15 to 45 minutes.

2. To serve, arrange melon wedges upright on individual plates and sprinkle each with a pinch of salt. Spoon strawberries and some juice over wedges and serve immediately.

TABLE TALK

Serve this as a delicious side dish for breakfast, lunch, or dinner, or have it on its own as a snack.

Cherries with Apricots and Lime

Lime and a trace of honey flavor a cherry sauce that's served with fresh apricots.

Yield:	Prep time:	Cook time:	Serving size:
6 cups	15 minutes	3 minutes	1 cup

Each serving has:				
88 calories	0.1 g total fat	0 g saturated fat	0 mg cholesterol	11 mg sodium
21.8 g carbohydrates	0.9 g fiber	5.1 g sugars	0.6 g protein	

1 tsp. lime zest	¾ lb. cherries, pitted and halved
2 TB. lime juice	4 ripe apricots, pitted and quartered
1 TB. honey	

1. In a medium saucepan, place the lime zest and juice with honey and about half of the cherries.

2. Bring to a boil over medium heat, stirring frequently. Reduce the heat to low and simmer, stirring constantly, until cherries are soft, about 3 minutes.

3. Remove the pan from heat and add remaining cherries. Set aside to cool or transfer to a bowl, cover, and refrigerate for up to 4 hours before serving.

4. Put apricots in a large bowl and add cooled cherry mixture. Toss until blended. Serve immediately in 4 small dessert bowls, or cover and refrigerate for up to 1 day before serving.

HEALTHY NOTE

A small amount of honey in a fruit side-dish recipe enhances the natural flavor of the fruit without changing the anti-inflammatory nature of the recipe. You can omit the honey, if you prefer, and you'll still enjoy the wonderful sweet taste of the fruit.

Red Grape Chutney

A sweet and tangy chutney holds the flavors of basil, oregano, and walnuts.

Yield:	Prep time:	Cook time:	Serving size:
5 cups	10 minutes	3 minutes	Scant ¼ cup

Each serving has:				
31 calories	1.3 g total fat	0 g saturated fat	1 mg cholesterol	4 mg sodium
5 g carbohydrates	0 g fiber	4.1 g sugars	0.5 g protein	

4 cups red seedless grapes (about 1¼ lb.)

1 TB. butter

½ cup red onion, chopped

¼ tsp. dried basil, crushed

¼ tsp. dried oregano, crushed

2 TB. red wine vinegar

¼ cup walnuts, chopped

1. Place grapes in a food processor. Process for 3 or 4 pulses until chopped. Set aside.

2. In a large skillet, melt butter. Add onion and cook until barely tender. Add basil and oregano, and cook for 1 minute. Add chopped grapes, vinegar, and walnuts. Cook 1 to 2 minutes more until heated through. Serve immediately.

HEALTHY NOTE

This tangy yet sweet chutney contains no added sugars, yet adds sparkle to your main-dish entrées. It tastes delicious as a side dish for pork tenderloin, grilled chicken, or seafood.

Blueberry Cheese Quesadillas

The fresh, sparkling taste of blueberries is accented with cream cheese on corn tortillas.

Yield:	Prep time:	Cook time:	Serving size:
8 quesadillas	15 minutes	8 to 10 minutes	1 quesadilla

Each serving has:				
138 calories	5.3 g total fat	1 g saturated fat	14 mg cholesterol	98 mg sodium
22 g carbohydrates	3.3 g fiber	8.8 g sugars	3.3 g protein	

8 6-in. corn tortillas	1 cup fresh or frozen blueberries, defrosted
1 TB. butter, melted	
4-oz. low-fat cream cheese, cut in 8 (¼-in.-thick) slices	1 cup fresh or frozen raspberries, defrosted

1. Preheat oven to 400°F.

2. Brush one side of each tortilla with melted butter. Place tortillas, buttered sides down, on a large baking sheet.

3. Place cheese slices on one half of each tortilla. Sprinkle blueberries over cheese. Fold other half of each tortilla over blueberries. Bake for 8 to 10 minutes or until golden brown and cheese is melted.

4. Meanwhile, place raspberries in a food processor. Cover and process until smooth. Serve quesadillas with raspberry sauce.

Variation: Substitute strawberries or cherries for the fruit in this recipe.

HEALTHY NOTE

Corn tortillas are made from ground corn, salt, and water. As such, they are an all-natural grain product.

Grilled Avocados

Grilled avocados hold spicy picante sauce and mild Monterey Jack cheese.

Yield:	Prep time:	Cook time:	Serving size:
4 avocado halves	10 minutes	10 minutes	1 half avocado

Each serving has:				
185 calories	15.4 g total fat	2.5 g saturated fat	1 mg cholesterol	131 mg sodium
11.1 g carbohydrates	7.5 g fiber	2.2 g sugars	4.4 g protein	

1 TB. lime juice

2 large ripe avocados, halved, seeded, and peeled (about 1 lb.)

¼ cup bottled picante sauce

1 oz. Monterey Jack or farmer cheese, shredded or crumbled (¼ cup)

2 TB. fresh cilantro, chopped

4 cups iceberg lettuce, shredded

1. Heat grill to medium. Brush lime juice over all sides of avocados.

2. Grill avocado halves uncovered, cut sides down, for 5 minutes or until browned. Turn avocado halves cut sides up. Fill each avocado half with 1 tablespoon picante sauce and 1 tablespoon shredded cheese. Cover grill and cook about 5 minutes more until cheese begins to melt.

3. Remove avocados from grill. Sprinkle tops of avocado halves with cilantro. Serve on a bed of salad greens.

TABLE TALK

Serve these spicy avocado halves with grilled meat or seafood, or with a South-of-the-Border-inspired main dish.

Banana Skillet

Enjoy the very sweet taste of sautéed bananas with bursts of flavor from oranges and earthy pecans.

Yield:	Prep time:	Cook time:	Serving size:
5 cups	15 minutes	5 to 10 minutes	⅝ cup

Each serving has:				
102 calories	5.7 g total fat	2.6 g saturated fat	4 mg cholesterol	12 mg sodium
13.4 g carbohydrates	2.6 g fiber	8.4 g sugars	1.2 g protein	

1 TB. butter	¼ cup pecans, toasted and chopped
2 medium bananas, sliced into ½-in. coins	½ cup unsweetened shredded coconut
2 medium oranges, peeled and sectioned	

1. Melt butter in a large skillet on medium heat. Add bananas, oranges, and pecans, and sauté gently for 5 to 10 minutes until bananas are fragrant but not mushy.

2. To serve, spoon warm fruit with juice into 8 small bowls. Top with coconut and serve immediately while warm.

TABLE TALK

Sautéing fruit in a small amount of butter brings out the flavor yet keeps the dish pro-health and anti-inflammatory.

Spicy Fruit Salsa

Sweet fresh fruit is marinated and flavored with cilantro, jalapeño, and lime juice to make a salsa or a side dish.

Yield:	Prep time:	Cook time:	Serving size:
4 cups	5 minutes plus 30 minutes chill time	None	¼ cup

Each serving has:

36 calories	2 g total fat	0 g saturated fat	0 mg cholesterol	36 mg sodium
4.9 g carbohydrates	1.4 g fiber	3 g sugars	0.6 g protein	

2 large nectarines, pitted and chopped

1 medium avocado, halved, seeded, peeled, and chopped

2 medium apricots, pitted and chopped

2 medium plums, pitted and chopped

¼ cup fresh cilantro, chopped

1 medium jalapeño pepper, seeded and finely chopped

2 TB. lime juice

1 tsp. garlic, minced

⅛ tsp. salt

1. In a medium bowl, combine nectarines, avocado, apricots, plums, cilantro, jalapeño pepper, lime juice, garlic, and salt. Cover and chill for at least 30 minutes before serving.

TABLE TALK

Chilling the salsa gives the ingredients the opportunity to blend and deliver more taste impact. Try serving it as a condiment with tortilla chips, fish, pork, or chicken.

Balsamic Berries with Cream

Fresh berries are wrapped in creamy, low-fat cheese and flavored with balsamic vinegar and vanilla.

Yield:	Prep time:	Cook time:	Serving size:
7 cups	35 minutes	None	⅞ cup

Each serving has:				
111 calories	5.6 g total fat	3.3 g saturated fat	17 mg cholesterol	101 mg sodium
12.2 g carbohydrates	3.4 g fiber	7.6 g sugars	4 g protein	

4 cups fresh strawberries, sliced

2 cups fresh blackberries

1 TB. honey

2 TB. balsamic vinegar

½ pkg. (8-oz.) reduced-fat cream cheese, softened

½ cup low-fat cottage cheese

1 tsp. vanilla extract

1. In a large bowl, combine strawberries, blackberries, honey, and balsamic vinegar. Cover and let stand for 30 minutes.

2. Meanwhile, in a large bowl, beat cream cheese, cottage cheese, and vanilla extract with an electric mixer on medium speed until smooth.

3. To serve, spoon berries into 8 small bowls and top with cream cheese mixture.

HEALTHY NOTE

Choose real vanilla extract and avoid imitation vanilla flavoring. There is a distinct difference—the extract tastes much better and imparts a fuller flavor. Imitation vanilla contains potentially inflammatory additives.

Golden Raisin and Eggplant Relish

This relish brings together the flavors of sweet raisins, spicy jalapeños, and tangy vinegar. Use it on main-course meat entrées or with eggs and cheese.

Yield:	Prep time:	Cook time:	Serving size:
3 cups	30 minutes	1½ hours	¼ cup

Each serving has:				
58 calories	3.5 g total fat	0 g saturated fat	0 mg cholesterol	53 mg sodium
6.5 g carbohydrates	1.9 g fiber	3.7 g sugars	0.8 g protein	

¼ cup golden raisins

3 TB. cider vinegar

1 eggplant (about 1½ lb.)

1 medium yellow onion, chopped

1 green or red bell pepper, cored, seeded, and chopped

3 TB. olive oil

1 jalapeño pepper, seeded and finely chopped

1½ tsp. garlic, minced

¼ tsp. salt

¼ tsp. freshly ground black pepper

1 medium tomato, chopped

2 TB. fresh Italian (flat-leaf) parsley, finely chopped

1. Preheat oven to 350°F. In a saucepan, combine raisins and vinegar. Bring to a boil. Remove from heat, cover, and set aside.

2. With the tip of a knife, pierce eggplant in five or six places. Place on foil-lined 15×10×1-inch baking pan. Roast for 1 to 1½ hours or until eggplant is soft to touch and collapsing. Remove from oven and cool. When cool enough to handle, cut eggplant in half lengthwise and scoop out flesh. Coarsely chop flesh and set aside.

3. In a medium skillet, cook onion and bell pepper in hot oil for 5 minutes or until tender. Stir in jalapeño, garlic, salt, and pepper. Cook, stirring often, for 3 minutes.

4. Stir raisin-vinegar mixture, eggplant, and tomato into the skillet. Bring to a low simmer and cook 5 minutes. Cover and refrigerate at least 8 hours or overnight.

5. To serve, let stand at room temperature 30 minutes. Stir in parsley. Serve with toasted baguette slices or as a relish over cheese, salmon, or chicken.

TABLE TALK

The golden raisins add natural sweetness to the tangy and savory eggplant relish. Try using this with scrambled eggs, or as a topping for fruit or steamed vegetables.

Orange Cranberry Salad

Serve this salad during the holidays in place of high-sugar cranberry sauce. It offers more flavor, too, with onion, ginger, and basil.

Yield:	Prep time:	Cook time:	Serving size:
8 cups	25 minutes	None	1 cup

Each serving has:				
75 calories	1.4 g total fat	0 g saturated fat	0 mg cholesterol	9 mg sodium
15.5 g carbohydrates	3.9 g fiber	10.3 g sugars	2 g protein	

2 cups fresh or frozen cranberries, thawed	2 TB. lemon juice
4 medium oranges, peeled	1 tsp. fresh ginger, grated
2 stalks celery, thinly sliced (1 cup)	1 (5-oz.) package arugula
¼ cup red onion, finely chopped	¼ cup fresh basil leaves, chopped
	2 TB. walnut oil

1. Place cranberries in food processor and pulse 5 times to chop coarsely. Transfer to a medium bowl.

2. Supreme oranges by removing the segments from the membrane over cranberry bowl to catch sections and juice. Stir in celery, onion, lemon juice, and ginger. Cover the bowl and refrigerate at least 1 hour or up to 2 days.

3. Toss arugula with basil and walnut oil. Top with cranberry mixture. Serve immediately.

TAKE CARE

Walnut oil is high in omega-3 fatty acids and adds rich taste to this salad. Don't use walnut oil for heating or sautéing, though. It loses its healthful qualities when heated, and your results would be disappointing.

Spicy Apple and Jicama Salad

Crisp jicama and apples are blended in yogurt with spicy chili powder and ginger.

Yield:	Prep time:	Cook time:	Serving size:
8 cups	15 minutes	None	$\frac{4}{5}$ cup

Each serving has:				
100 calories	2.3 g total fat	0 g saturated fat	1 mg cholesterol	18 mg sodium
19.1 g carbohydrates	3.1 g fiber	14.2 g sugars	2.3 g protein	

1 (6-oz.) carton plain low-fat yogurt

1 tsp. chili powder

2 TB. candied ginger, finely chopped

3 medium apples, cored and cut into bite-size pieces

2 cups jicama, chopped

2 cups red seedless grapes, halved

$\frac{1}{2}$ cup fresh or frozen cherries, thawed, pitted, and halved

$\frac{1}{4}$ cup walnuts, toasted and chopped

1. In a large bowl, combine yogurt, chili powder, and ginger. Stir until well combined. Add apple, jicama, grapes, and cherries. Toss to coat.

2. Cover and chill 1 hour. To serve, top with walnuts.

TABLE TALK

Chili powder gives a hot bite to this crunchy salad. You can vary the amount of chili powder based on how much heat you want.

Nectarine Salad

Nectarines are in the dressing, along with fresh rosemary, Dijon mustard, and walnut oil. They're also an ingredient in the salad, along with raspberries and pine nuts. Scrumptious!

Yield:	Prep time:	Cook time:	Serving size:
12 cups	20 minutes	None	2 cups

Each serving has:				
165 calories	7.4 g total fat	0.6 g saturated fat	0 mg cholesterol	163 mg sodium
24.7 g carbohydrates	6.2 g fiber	15.6 g sugars	4.6 g protein	

7 medium fresh nectarines, pitted and halved	½ tsp. salt
2 TB. water	¼ tsp. freshly ground black pepper
2 TB. plus 2 tsp. fresh rosemary	6 cups mixed salad greens, torn
3 TB. lemon juice	1 cup fresh or frozen raspberries, defrosted
2 TB. Dijon-style mustard	¼ cup pine nuts, toasted
3 TB. walnut oil	

1. Coarsely chop 1 nectarine and place in a food processor with water, 2 tablespoons rosemary, lemon juice, mustard, oil, salt, and pepper.

2. Slice remaining nectarines. In a very large salad bowl combine sliced nectarines, greens, and raspberries. Drizzle with dressing and toss to coat.

3. Divide salad among 6 salad plates. Sprinkle with pine nuts and remaining 2 teaspoons snipped rosemary.

TABLE TALK

Toasting pine nuts intensifies their flavor, browns them, and makes them crunchier. Place nuts in a dry skillet over medium-low heat. Shake the skillet frequently to ensure even browning, watching carefully, as they could burn. When the nuts are light brown and fragrant, remove to a bowl or plate to cool.

Vegetable Side Dishes

Chapter

15

In This Chapter

- Cooking vegetables to preserve anti-inflammatory nutrients
- Unique combinations of vegetables and flavorings
- Enjoying time-tested vegetable favorites
- Adding healthy fat to vegetables for higher nutrient absorption

Vegetables are a keystone in healthy eating and reducing inflammation, so eat lots of them. You can't go wrong eating green vegetables. Experts recommend eating 5 to 10 daily servings of vegetables/fruit, specifically eating 1 to 3 servings of fruit, and 4 to 9 servings of vegetables. Yes, you read that correctly. That's three servings per meal, with one left over for a snack.

If we all ate our recommended daily vegetable/fruit servings, fewer folks would be overweight and type 2 diabetes would be a thing of the past. Perhaps most heart disease, arthritis, and other chronic health concerns and autoimmune disorders would also be a thing of the past. Why? Because we'd all have far less inflammation.

To eat this well and this opulently, you need many choices. That's why we've written 25 vegetable recipes for you to choose from. So choose many and choose often.

Be sure to purchase organic produce when you can. The organic versions don't necessarily have more nutrients, but overall, they have fewer toxins than those conventionally grown. This translates into a reduction in inflammatory components in your vegetables.

We didn't include recipes for white potatoes, such as baked potatoes or french fries, in this chapter. They are high-glycemic and increase inflammation rather than reduce it. Instead, you'll find recipes for low-glycemic yams. They offer more flavor and are cooked in similar ways.

Spicy Collard Greens

These greens give you a healthful taste of the South—they're flavored with turkey bacon, molasses, and hot pepper sauce.

Yield:	Prep time:	Cook time:	Serving size:
4 cups	10 minutes	7 to 8 hours	½ cup

Each serving has:				
55 calories	1.1 g total fat	0 g saturated fat	4 mg cholesterol	140 mg sodium
10 g carbohydrates	4 g fiber	2 g sugars	3.9 g protein	

2 lb. collard greens, trimmed and coarsely torn

1 large yellow onion, chopped

4 tsp. garlic, minced

3 slices extra-lean turkey bacon, coarsely chopped

1 TB. light or dark molasses

2 TB. balsamic vinegar

1 tsp. bottled hot pepper sauce

1 tsp. celery seeds

3½ cups water

¼ tsp. salt

¼ tsp. freshly ground black pepper

1. Place greens, onion, garlic, bacon, molasses, vinegar, pepper sauce, celery seeds, water, salt, and pepper in a 5- or 6-quart slow cooker. Cover and cook on the low heat setting for 7 to 8 hours, stirring once after 4 hours of cooking.

2. Using a slotted spoon, transfer greens to a serving dish, reserving cooking liquid. If desired, spoon some cooking liquid over each serving.

TABLE TALK

Molasses is a syrup directly derived from sugar cane, making it a natural form of sugar.

Asparagus with Citrus

Asparagus spears are baked on a bed of orange and lemon slices, and then finished with garlic and tarragon for a delightful taste.

Yield:	Prep time:	Cook time:	Serving size:
2 pounds	15 minutes	12 minutes	¼ pound

Each serving has:				
124 calories	8.7 g total fat	0 g saturated fat	0 g trans fat	0 mg cholesterol
77 mg sodium	11.4 g carbohydrates	3.9 g fiber	6.8 g sugars	3.1 g protein

2 medium oranges	2 tsp. fresh tarragon leaves or 1 tsp. dried
2 medium lemons	¼ tsp. salt
5 TB. olive oil	¼ tsp. freshly ground black pepper
2 lb. asparagus, trimmed	
2 cloves garlic, thinly sliced	

1. Preheat oven to 400°F. From one orange and one lemon, cut ⅛×2-inch strips of the zest, avoiding bitter white pith (about 10 to 16 strips). Squeeze orange and lemon to obtain 2 tablespoons juice.

2. Peel remaining orange and lemon. Thinly slice orange and lemon and toss with 1 tablespoon of olive oil. Place on a baking sheet lined with parchment paper.

3. Place asparagus spears in a separate 15×10×1-inch baking pan. Sprinkle with garlic, tarragon, and citrus zest strips. Drizzle with 2 tablespoons of olive oil and toss to coat. Spread in a single layer in the pan.

4. Roast asparagus and citrus slices, in separate pans, 12 to 15 minutes, turning once or twice with tongs, until asparagus is tender and citrus begins to brown. Transfer asparagus mixture to a serving platter.

5. Meanwhile, for vinaigrette, in a small bowl, whisk together reserved fruit juice, remaining 2 tablespoons oil, salt, and pepper.

6. Drizzle vinaigrette over roasted asparagus, citrus zest, and garlic. Sprinkle with roasted citrus slices. Serve warm.

TABLE TALK

Trim asparagus by breaking off the woody bottoms of each stalk.

Honey Roasted Broccoli

Broccoli is baked with a breadcrumb mixture flavored with honey and mustard.

Yield:	Prep time:	Cook time:	Serving size:
8 cups	10 minutes	17-20 minutes	1 cup

Each serving has:				
136 calories	7.5 g total fat	2.4 g saturated fat	8 mg cholesterol	118 mg sodium
15.7 g carbohydrates	2.9 g fiber	6.3 g sugars	3.7 g protein	

2 TB. honey	⅓ cup fresh parsley, chopped
2 TB. whole-grain mustard	2 whole heads broccoli, trimmed and cut into pieces
2 TB. olive oil	
½ cup fresh whole-wheat breadcrumbs	

1. Preheat oven to 400°F. Combine honey, mustard, olive oil, breadcrumbs, and parsley in a small bowl. Set aside.

2. Place broccoli in a vegetable steamer and steam for 3 to 5 minutes, until al dente. Remove to a large bowl. Coat broccoli with breadcrumb mixture. Place broccoli in a large baking dish and bake 12 to 15 minutes or until broccoli heads are tender.

3. Remove from oven and place broccoli on a serving platter. Serve hot.

TABLE TALK

Make your own breadcrumbs by processing day-old stone-ground bread in the food processor. You can also substitute almond or pecan flour for the breadcrumbs.

Green Beans with Basil

Green beans are flavored with a combination of garlic, basil, mint, and yellow bell pepper.

Yield:	Prep time:	Cook time:	Serving size:
8 cups	10 minutes	7 minutes	1 cup

Each serving has:				
70 calories	3.6 g total fat	0.5 g saturated fat	0 mg cholesterol	156 mg sodium
9 g carbohydrates	4.3 g fiber	2 g sugars	2.3 g protein	

2 lb. fresh green beans, trimmed	1 small yellow bell pepper, cored, seeded, and chopped
¼ tsp. garlic, minced	2 TB. olive oil
½ cup shredded fresh basil	½ tsp. salt
⅓ cup shredded fresh mint	

1. In a vegetable steamer, steam beans until al dente, 2 to 4 minutes.

2. Meanwhile, in a large bowl, combine garlic, basil, mint, bell pepper, olive oil, and salt. Add drained green beans. Toss gently to combine.

TABLE TALK

The portions of basil and mint in this recipe may be larger than you'd expect. This quantity of fresh herbs gives a sparkling flavor to the beans and provides plenty of powerful antioxidants.

Celery Root Cakes with Yams

Add these vegetable cakes to any meal—you'll get raves for the unique flavor of toasted cumin seeds.

Yield:	Prep time:	Cook time:	Serving size:
16 cakes	30 minutes	5 minutes	2 cakes

Each serving has:				
148 calories	9.7 g total fat	1.6 g saturated fat	47 mg cholesterol	147 mg sodium
13 g carbohydrates	2.2 g fiber	3.5 g sugars	2.9 g protein	

1½ tsp. cumin seeds	12 oz. celery root, peeled and shredded
5 TB. olive oil	
2 large eggs, slightly beaten	12 oz. yams (2 small), peeled and shredded
2 tsp. garlic, minced	
¼ tsp. salt	

1. In a small, dry skillet, toast cumin seeds over medium heat for 2 to 3 minutes or until lightly toasted. Remove from heat. Cool seeds and crush slightly with a mortar and pestle.

2. In a large bowl, whisk together 3 tablespoons olive oil, eggs, garlic, salt, and crushed cumin seeds. Stir in celery root and yams until combined. Form mixture into 16 cakes, stirring mixture frequently to keep egg mixture well distributed.

3. In a large skillet, heat 1 tablespoon of olive oil over medium-high heat. Add 6 to 8 cakes to the pan and cook for 5 to 6 minutes or until cakes are golden brown, turning once. Repeat with remaining vegetable mixture, adding additional oil as needed during cooking. If necessary, reduce heat to medium to prevent over-browning. Drain on paper towels.

4. Serve at once, or refrigerate and serve at room temperature. Will keep in refrigerator for one week.

TABLE TALK

Shred the celery root and yams with a food processor or with a hand-held grater.

Butternut Squash Bake

Curry and olive oil flavors the baked squash. Serve on skewers for a squash kabob.

Yield:	Prep time:	Cook time:	Serving size:
1 squash	15 minutes	20 to 25 minutes	$\frac{1}{8}$ squash

Each serving has:				
94 calories	5 g total fat	1.4 g saturated fat	4 mg cholesterol	15 mg sodium
13.4 g carbohydrates	2.4 g fiber	2.5 g sugars	1.2 g protein	

1 2-lb. butternut squash	2 TB. olive oil
1 TB. butter, melted	1 tsp. curry powder

1. Preheat oven to 450°F. Cut squash in half lengthwise and remove seeds. Peel squash. Cut squash halves in 1- to $1\frac{1}{2}$-inch pieces. Place in a 3-quart rectangular baking dish.

2. In a small bowl, combine butter, oil, and curry powder. Drizzle over squash, tossing to coat.

3. Roast squash, uncovered, for 20 to 25 minutes or until tender and lightly browned, stirring once or twice. Serve immediately or let cool to make kabobs.

4. To make kabobs, serve squash at room temperature threaded on eight 8-inch skewers. Store in an airtight container in the refrigerator up to 2 days.

 HEALTHY NOTE

The curry adds so much flavor to the squash that this dish doesn't require additional salt.

Cauliflower with Pine Nuts

Flax seeds and pine nuts top this cauliflower-and-ham duo.

Yield:	Prep time:	Cook time:	Serving size:
12 wedges	10 minutes	7 to 9 minutes	2 wedges

Each serving has:				
120 calories	8.2 g total fat	1.4 g saturated fat	7 mg cholesterol	199 mg sodium
6.4 g carbohydrates	2.7 g fiber	2.4 g sugars	6.7 g protein	

2 small heads cauliflower

2 oz. Serrano ham, cooked ham, or prosciutto, thinly sliced

2 oz. low-fat Monterey Jack cheese, shredded

¼ cup olive oil

2 TB. lemon juice

1 tsp. garlic, minced

¼ tsp. freshly ground black pepper

2 TB. toasted pine nuts

1 TB. flax seeds

1. Remove heavy leaves and tough stems from cauliflower; cut into 6 wedges. Place cauliflower in a vegetable steamer. Bring water to boiling and steam for 7 to 9 minutes or just until tender.

2. Divide ham slices equally among 6 serving plates. Divide cauliflower wedges among serving plates. Sprinkle with cheese.

3. In a screw-top jar, combine oil, lemon juice, garlic, and pepper. Shake well to combine. Drizzle over cauliflower, ham, and cheese. Sprinkle with pine nuts and flax seeds.

HEALTHY NOTE

This recipe doesn't include salt because the cheese and ham add plenty of salt to the recipe.

Roasted Basil Tomatoes

This simple dish of baked tomatoes will delight your taste buds with the fragrant flavor of basil and olive oil.

Yield:	Prep time:	Cook time:	Serving size:
16 halves	20 minutes	45 minutes	2⅔ halves

Each serving has:				
53 calories	3.2 g total fat	0 g saturated fat	0 mg cholesterol	112 mg sodium
5.8 g carbohydrates	1.3 g fiber	4.5 g sugars	1.4 g protein	

8 plum tomatoes (1½ lb.)	¼ tsp. salt
4 tsp. olive oil	¼ tsp. freshly ground black pepper
3 TB. fresh basil, chopped, or 1 TB. dried basil leaves	Fresh basil (optional)

1. Preheat oven to 375°F. Halve tomatoes lengthwise. Scoop out seeds and center membranes. Place tomatoes in a shallow roasting pan, cut sides up. Drizzle with oil.

2. In a small bowl, combine chopped basil, salt, and pepper. Sprinkle mixture over tomatoes.

3. Roast tomatoes, uncovered, for 45 minutes. Remove from oven. If desired, sprinkle with fresh basil. Serve warm.

HEALTHY NOTE

Baking vegetables retains the vitamins and minerals that can be washed out when they are boiled in water.

Roasted Italian Vegetables

Roasted garlic cloves, along with rosemary and oregano, add flavor to the vegetables.

Yield:	Prep time:	Cook time:	Serving size:
6 cups	15 minutes	35 to 40 minutes	1 cup

Each serving has:

157 calories	9.5 g total fat	1.3 g saturated fat	0 mg cholesterol	167 mg sodium
17.3 g carbohydrates	4.9 g fiber	6.3 g sugars	2.9 g protein	

¾ lb. carrots, cut into 3-in. pieces

1 large red bell pepper, cored, seeded, and cut into ½-in.-wide pieces

1 large yellow bell pepper, cored, seeded, and cut into ½-in.-wide pieces

1 large fennel bulb, cut into 6 wedges

1 medium red onion, cut into eighths

1 head garlic, divided into unpeeled cloves

2 sprigs fresh rosemary

2 sprigs fresh oregano

4 TB. olive oil

¼ tsp. salt

¼ tsp. freshly ground black pepper

2 small zucchini, cut into 1-in. rounds

1. Preheat oven to 400°F.

2. On a rimmed baking sheet, toss carrots, bell peppers, fennel, onion, garlic, rosemary, and oregano with 3 tablespoons olive oil. Sprinkle with salt and pepper. Roast for 15 minutes.

3. Meanwhile, in a small bowl, toss zucchini with remaining 1 tablespoon olive oil.

4. Add zucchini to the baking sheet and toss. Continue roasting for 20 to 25 more minutes, until vegetables are tender.

5. Remove from the oven and squeeze roasted garlic cloves from their skins onto vegetables and toss well to distribute. Serve at once.

TABLE TALK

Garlic roasted in this way becomes mild and has a sweet taste. If you find that you like roasted garlic, use it as a spread for crackers or crostini.

Root Vegetable Roast

This plethora of nutrition gives you flavorful vegetables seasoned with garlic, thyme, and paprika.

Yield:	Prep time:	Cook time:	Serving size:
16 cups	10 minutes	30 minutes	2 cups

Each serving has:				
269 calories	7.2 g total fat	1 g saturated fat	0 mg cholesterol	140 mg sodium
49.4 g carbohydrates	9 g fiber	8.1 g sugars	3.5 g protein	

2 medium golden beets, peeled	$\frac{1}{4}$ cup olive oil
2 medium white turnips, unpeeled	3 TB. dried thyme
2 medium yams, unpeeled	4 cloves garlic, peeled and sliced
2 medium carrots, peeled	$\frac{1}{4}$ tsp. salt
2 medium parsnips, peeled	$\frac{1}{4}$ tsp. paprika
2 small yellow onions	

1. Preheat oven to 400°F.

2. Cut beets and turnips into 6 wedges each. Cut yams in half crosswise, then into 6 wedges, for a total of 12 wedges for each yam. Halve carrots and parsnips lengthwise and then crosswise. Cut onions into quarters.

3. In a small skillet, combine oil, thyme, and garlic. Simmer over low heat for 5 minutes. Remove from heat.

4. In a large bowl, toss vegetables with oil mixture. Transfer to a large baking pan and arrange in an even layer. Roast for 15 minutes.

5. Roast for 30 minutes, turning vegetables once, until tender. Transfer vegetables to a serving platter. Season with salt and paprika. Serve warm.

TABLE TALK

This is a delicious and simple way to sample the taste and goodness of winter vegetables.

Roasted Garlic

Slow-roasted garlic is surprisingly sweet and mild, and highly satisfying to the palate.

Yield:	Prep time:	Cook time:	Serving size:
8 garlic heads	5 minutes	30 to 35 minutes	1 garlic head

Each serving has:				
76 calories	4.6 g total fat	0.6 g saturated fat	0 mg cholesterol	4 mg sodium
7.9 g carbohydrates	0.5 g fiber	0 g sugars	1.5 g protein	

8 heads garlic	8 tsp. olive oil

1. Preheat oven to 400°F.

2. Peel away outer layers of garlic bulbs, leaving skins of individual cloves intact. Using a knife, cut off ¼ to ½ inch of the top of each clove, exposing the individual cloves of garlic.

3. Place each garlic head in a muffin pan space. Drizzle 1 teaspoon of olive oil over each head, using your fingers to make sure garlic head is well coated. Cover with aluminum foil and bake for 30 to 35 minutes. Remove and let garlic sit until it is cool to the touch.

4. Squeeze each garlic clove out of its skin. Eat as is, or spread on vegetable scoopers, crostini, bread, or crackers. You can refrigerate for later use in salads, in salad dressings, and as a garnish for meat or vegetables.

TABLE TALK

Serve this very simple recipe as an appetizer. Folks will enjoy squeezing out the garlic cloves. Provide a colorful assortment of vegetable scoopers, such as cucumber wheels, carrot sticks, cauliflower florets, and bell pepper sticks.

Green Beans with Walnuts and Salmon

Salmon adds protein and flavor to green beans that are topped with walnuts.

Yield:	Prep time:	Cook time:	Serving size:
8 cups	10 minutes	3 to 5 minutes	1 cup

Each serving has:				
148 calories	10.5 g total fat	1.1 g saturated fat	3 mg cholesterol	313 mg sodium
9.1 g carbohydrates	4.2 g fiber	2.2 g sugars	6.5 g protein	

3 (9-oz.) packages frozen whole green beans	½ cup red onion, chopped
1 large red bell pepper, cored, seeded, and cut into thin strips	3 TB. olive oil
	3 TB. red wine vinegar
1 (4-oz.) package cracked-pepper smoked salmon, skinned and broken into chunks	1 TB. Dijon-style mustard
	1 tsp. garlic, minced
	½ cup walnuts, coarsely chopped

1. In a vegetable steamer, cook beans for 3 to 5 minutes or until crisp-tender.

2. In a large bowl, combine beans, bell pepper, salmon, and red onion.

3. In a small bowl, whisk together olive oil, vinegar, mustard, and garlic. Add to bean mixture and toss to coat.

4. Divide bean mixture among 8 side plates or transfer to a serving dish. Top with walnuts. Serve hot or cold.

HEALTHY NOTE

Smoked salmon is an excellent addition to cooked vegetables. Along with the walnuts, it provides important omega-3 fatty acids.

Baked Acorn Squash

Fragrant pine nuts and maple syrup fill the centers of acorn squash, bringing an earthy autumn taste to the meal.

Yield:	Prep time:	Cook time:	Serving size:
6 halves	10 minutes	1 hour	1 half

Each serving has:				
261 calories	16.3 g total fat	3.7 g saturated fat	10 mg cholesterol	35 mg sodium
30.3 g carbohydrates	3.8 g fiber	5.7 g sugars	3.6 g protein	

3 medium acorn squash	2 TB. maple syrup
$\frac{1}{2}$ cup pine nuts	$\frac{1}{2}$ tsp. cinnamon
2 TB. butter	$\frac{1}{2}$ tsp. ground ginger
2 TB. olive oil	$\frac{1}{4}$ tsp. nutmeg (optional)

1. Preheat oven to 375°F.

2. Cut each squash in half lengthwise and scoop out seeds.

3. Arrange squash halves in an 11×15-inch shallow baking pan. Into each depression, place $\frac{1}{6}$ of pine nuts, 1 teaspoon butter, 1 teaspoon olive oil, and 1 teaspoon maple syrup. Sprinkle each evenly with cinnamon and ginger. Bake for 1 hour or until tender.

4. Serve warm. Sprinkle with nutmeg, if desired.

TABLE TALK

Even folks who eschew vegetables fall in culinary love with baked acorn squash. It contains plentiful beta-carotene and antioxidants.

Yam Fries

Yams come out of the oven steamy and sweet with the fragrant flavor of rosemary.

Yield:	Prep time:	Cook time:	Serving size:
6 cups	15 minutes	25 minutes	1 cup

Each serving has:				
234 calories	6.7 g total fat	1.9 g saturated fat	5 mg cholesterol	221 mg sodium
41.9 g carbohydrates	6.2 g fiber	0.8 g sugars	236 g protein	

1 TB. butter	3 medium yams
2 TB. olive oil	½ tsp. salt
2 TB. dried rosemary	¼ tsp. freshly ground black pepper

1. Preheat oven to 450°F.

2. In a small saucepan, melt butter with olive oil over medium heat. Stir in rosemary.

3. Cut yams lengthwise into 1½-inch-thick wedges and place in a large bowl. Drizzle with rosemary mixture. Toss gently.

4. Arrange yam wedges in a single layer so they don't touch on a large baking sheet lined in aluminum foil. Bake in the upper third of the oven for 20 minutes, turning once, or until softened and lightly browned. Season with salt and pepper. Serve warm.

TABLE TALK

Serve these as a more healthful and tastier alternative to french fries.

Pearl Onions Italiano

The sweetness of pearl onions is accented with vinegar and herbs.

Yield:	Prep time:	Cook time:	Serving size:
3 cups	10 minutes	6 to 7 minutes	¾ cup

Each serving has:				
60 calories	2 g total fat	1.2 g saturated fat	5 mg cholesterol	114 mg sodium
10 g carbohydrates	1.3 g fiber	6.1 g sugars	0.9 g protein	

1 lb. frozen pearl onions, thawed	1 TB. butter
1 TB. honey	2 TB. fresh parsley, chopped
¼ cup red wine vinegar	2 TB. fresh basil, chopped
¼ tsp. salt	

1. In a vegetable steamer, cook onions until al dente, about 2 minutes.

2. In a large skillet over medium heat, add onions, honey, and vinegar. Reduce to a simmer and cook until onions are tender, about 4 minutes. Remove from heat and stir in salt, butter, parsley, and basil.

TABLE TALK

This side dish of pearl onions adds flavor enhancement to entrées such as beef, lamb, and chicken dishes. Omit the honey, if you prefer. It enhances the sweetness of the onions.

Broccoli with Sunflower Seeds

Black olives and sunflower seeds impart crunch and color to Italian-flavored broccoli.

Yield:	Prep time:	Cook time:	Serving size:
4 cups	10 minutes	5 minutes	$\frac{2}{3}$ cup

Each serving has:				
97 calories	7.1 g total fat	0.9 g saturated fat	0 g cholesterol	148 mg sodium
7.3 mg carbohydrates	2.6 g fiber	1.9 g sugars	3.1 g protein	

1 lb. broccoli, cut into 1-in. pieces	2 TB. black olives, chopped
2 TB. olive oil	1$\frac{1}{2}$ tsp. Italian herb seasoning
1 small white onion, chopped	$\frac{1}{2}$ cup sunflower seeds, toasted
1 tsp. garlic, minced	$\frac{1}{4}$ tsp. salt
2 TB. fresh parsley, chopped	$\frac{1}{4}$ tsp. freshly ground black pepper

1. In a steamer, cook broccoli about 5 minutes until al dente.

2. In a large skillet, heat olive oil over medium heat. Add onion and garlic, and cook until softened. Stir in parsley, olives, Italian herb seasoning, and sunflower seeds.

3. Add cooked broccoli to skillet and season with salt and pepper. Toss to combine and serve hot.

TABLE TALK

If you choose not to use the broccoli stems, shred them in a food processor for later use in salads and soups.

Cabbage with Caraway

Caraway seed and horseradish offer a traditional Eastern Europe flavor to the cabbage.

Yield:	Prep time:	Cook time:	Serving size:
6 cups	10 minutes	5 minutes	¾ cup

Each serving has:				
62 calories	4.5 g total fat	2.8 g saturated fat	11 mg cholesterol	122 mg sodium
5.4 g carbohydrates	2.4 g fiber	2.9 g sugars	1.2 g protein	

1 head cabbage, shredded	1 tsp. caraway seeds
3 TB. butter, melted	¼ tsp. salt
1 tsp. white wine vinegar	¼ tsp. freshly ground black pepper
1 tsp. prepared horseradish	

1. In a steamer, cook cabbage until crisp-tender, about 5 minutes. Transfer to a serving dish.

2. In a small bowl, combine butter, vinegar, horseradish, and caraway seeds. Add mixture to cabbage, and toss. Season with salt and pepper.

HEALTHY NOTE

This recipe calls for butter because it imparts a creamy flavor to the cabbage. If you prefer to pass on the butter, substitute olive oil.

Celery Root Sauté

Celery root offers a light, creamy celery flavor that complements the carrot and garlic.

Yield:	Prep time:	Cook time:	Serving size:
4 cups	10 minutes	10 to 12 minutes	1 cup

Each serving has:				
115 calories	7.1 g total fat	1 g saturated fat	0 mg cholesterol	271 mg sodium
12.1 g carbohydrates	2.5 g fiber	2.5 g sugars	1.9 g protein	

2 TB. olive oil	1 tsp. garlic, minced
1 lb. celery root, peeled, halved, and cut into thick matchsticks	⅓ cup water
	1 tsp. celery seeds
1 carrot, cut into thick matchsticks	¼ tsp. salt

1. In a large skillet, heat oil over medium heat. Add celery root, carrot, and garlic, and cook, tossing frequently, until celery root is golden brown around the edges, about 7 minutes.

2. Add water and celery seeds to skillet and cook until celery root and carrot are crisp-tender and water has evaporated, 3 to 5 minutes. Season with salt.

TABLE TALK

Celery root, also known as celeriac, is a kind of celery that imparts a mild celery taste.

Roasted Fennel with Parmesan

Fennel lends a light hint of licorice flavor, made all the more delectable with a coating of Parmesan.

Yield:	Prep time:	Cook time:	Serving size:
4 cups	10 minutes	45 minutes	$\frac{2}{3}$ cup

Each serving has:				
113 calories	6.4 g total fat	1.6 g saturated fat	5 mg cholesterol	166 mg sodium
11.6 g carbohydrates	4.8 g fiber	0 g sugars	4.1 g protein	

4 bulbs fennel (1 lb. each), stalks discarded, cut into $\frac{1}{2}$-in. slices vertically

$\frac{1}{3}$ cup Parmesan cheese, grated

2 TB. olive oil

1 TB. balsamic vinegar

1. Preheat oven to 375°F.

2. Lightly oil the bottom of a 13×9×2-inch glass baking dish. Arrange fennel in the dish. Sprinkle with Parmesan and drizzle with olive oil.

3. Bake until fennel is fork-tender and top is golden brown, about 45 minutes.

4. Sprinkle with balsamic vinegar. Serve warm or cold.

TABLE TALK

Fennel imparts a sweet, slightly peppery and licorice taste, and is delicious combined with the tangy taste of cheese and balsamic vinegar. Often only the bulb is used in cooking.

Carrots with Hazelnuts and Lemon

Baby carrots are flavored with lemon, with added crunch and flavor from toasted hazelnuts.

Yield:	Prep time:	Cook time:	Serving size:
4 cups	10 minutes	5 minutes	⅔ cup

Each serving has:				
132 calories	8.5 g total fat	0.9 g saturated fat	0 g cholesterol	215 mg sodium
13.6 mg carbohydrates	5 g fiber	7.5 g sugars	1.9 g protein	

2 lb. baby carrots	Zest from 1 lemon, cut into thin strips
2 TB. olive oil	¼ tsp. salt
½ cup hazelnuts, coarsely chopped	¼ tsp. freshly ground black pepper

1. In a steamer, cook carrots about 5 minutes until al dente.

2. In a large skillet, heat olive oil over medium heat. Add hazelnuts and cook, stirring often, until lightly browned and toasted, 3 to 5 minutes. Stir in carrots and lemon zest. Sprinkle on salt and pepper. Toss to coat. Serve hot.

TABLE TALK

If you choose to use regular-size carrots, scrub or peel them and then slice into ⅜-inch coins.

Golden Beet Salad

This beautifully colored salad is tossed with a white wine vinaigrette dressing.

Yield:	Prep time:	Cook time:	Serving size:
8 cups	30 minutes	40 to 45 minutes	1 cup

Each serving has:				
164 calories	7.4 g total fat	0.9 g saturated fat	0 mg cholesterol	195 mg sodium
22.7 g carbohydrates	6.6 g fiber	13.2 g sugars	5 g protein	

12 golden beets, trimmed and cut into quarters	½ medium red onion, thinly sliced into half-circles
3 TB. olive oil	⅓ cup almonds, sliced and toasted
1½ lb. fresh green beans, trimmed	¼ tsp. salt
1 TB. orange juice	¼ tsp. freshly ground black pepper
1 TB. white wine vinegar	

1. Preheat oven to 400°F.

2. Place beets in a 3-quart rectangular baking dish. Drizzle beets with 1 table-spoon olive oil and toss lightly to coat. Cover dish with foil. Bake 40 to 45 minutes until tender.

3. Steam beans in a steamer basket in a covered saucepan over boiling water for 3 to 4 minutes. Remove basket from the saucepan and rinse under cold water. Place beans in a colander to drain.

4. In a small bowl, whisk together 2 tablespoons olive oil, orange juice, and vinegar.

5. In a serving bowl, add beets, beans, orange juice mixture, and onion. Toss gently. Fold in almonds and season with salt and pepper. Serve at room temperature.

TABLE TALK

If you're short on time, use 2 cans of sliced red beets instead of fresh beets. Be sure to drain them well before adding to salad.

Roasted Brussels Sprouts with Aioli

Chipotle chili with mayonnaise tops Brussels sprouts roasted with flavorful garlic and lemon.

Yield:	Prep time:	Cook time:	Serving size:
50 Brussels sprouts	15 minutes	17 to 20 minutes	About 25 half-sprouts

Each serving has:				
193 calories	9.4 g total fat	1.4 g saturated fat	4 mg cholesterol	232 mg sodium
24.3 g carbohydrates	5 g fiber	4.3 g sugars	5.9 g protein	

1 lb. small Brussels sprouts, trimmed	2 tsp. lemon zest
1 TB. olive oil	1 TB. garlic, minced
2 TB. lemon juice	¼ cup low-fat mayonnaise
½ cup panko	1 chipotle chile in adobo sauce, minced

1. Preheat oven to 400°F.

2. Cut Brussels sprouts in half lengthwise. Make a ½-inch cut into the stem of each sprout half so the stem cooks evenly.

3. Transfer Brussels sprouts to a large bowl and drizzle with olive oil and 1 table-spoon lemon juice. Sprinkle panko, 1 teaspoon lemon zest, and garlic over top of sprouts, and toss until lightly coated.

4. On a rimmed baking sheet, spread sprouts–panko mixture in an even layer. Roast in oven for 10 minutes. Remove from oven and use tongs to quickly turn sprouts over. Return to oven and bake until tender, 7 to 10 more minutes.

5. Meanwhile, prepare aioli: in a small bowl, whisk together mayonnaise, 1 table-spoon lemon juice, 1 teaspoon lemon zest, and chipotle chile.

6. Remove sprouts from the oven and place on a large serving platter. Serve aioli on the side for dipping.

TABLE TALK

Keep a can of chipotle chilies in adobo sauce in your pantry. They lend a hot, spicy, and smoky flavor to sauces, vegetables, tacos, and other South-of-the Border fare. Refrigerate in an airtight container after opening. Will keep in the refrigerator for 2 weeks.

Fennel and Yam Bake

Yam and fennel slices are layered with fragrant rosemary, garlic, and lemon.

Yield:	Prep time:	Cook time:	Serving size:
1 9×9-inch dish	15 minutes	1 hour	$\frac{1}{4}$ dish

Each serving has:				
74 calories	2.4 g total fat	0 g saturated fat	0 mg cholesterol	177 mg sodium
11.8 g carbohydrates	3.1 g fiber	2.1 g sugars	2.1 g protein	

1 large yam, unpeeled and cut into $\frac{1}{8}$-in. slices	1 medium fennel bulb, trimmed and cut into $\frac{1}{8}$-in. slices
2 tsp. olive oil	1 tsp. lemon zest
$\frac{1}{4}$ tsp. salt	2 TB. lemon juice
$\frac{1}{4}$ tsp. freshly ground black pepper	1 cup low-sodium chicken broth
4 sprigs fresh rosemary	3 green onions, thinly sliced
2 cloves garlic, thinly sliced	

1. Preheat oven to 375°F.

2. In a medium bowl, toss yams with olive oil and season with salt and pepper.

3. Lay rosemary sprigs in the bottom of a 9×9-inch baking dish. Scatter garlic over rosemary. Arrange alternating slices of yam and fennel in the dish until all vegetables are used, overlapping each slice.

4. Sprinkle vegetables with lemon zest and pour lemon juice and broth into the baking dish. Cover dish with foil and roast in the oven for 50 minutes or until yams are tender when pierced with a fork. Remove foil and continue to roast for another 6 to 8 minutes to allow yams to brown.

5. Remove dish from the oven. Transfer vegetables to a serving platter, discard rosemary, and drizzle all liquid from the dish over top. Sprinkle onions over top. Cut into 4 portions. Serve warm or cool.

TABLE TALK

If you don't have fresh rosemary on hand, use 4 teaspoons dried rosemary and scatter in between the yam and fennel layers.

Stuffed Portobello Mushrooms

Large mushrooms are stuffed with flavorful onions, garlic, and vegetables.

Yield:	Prep time:	Cook time:	Serving size:
4 stuffed mushrooms	15 minutes	24 minutes	1 stuffed mushroom

Each serving has:				
157 calories	5.5 g total fat	2.4 g saturated fat	11 mg cholesterol	370 mg sodium
17.4 g carbohydrates	3.4 g fiber	4.4 g sugars	10.6 g protein	

4 large portobello mushrooms	2 roasted red peppers, chopped
1 tsp. olive oil	$\frac{1}{2}$ cup fresh basil leaves, chopped
1 zucchini, chopped	$\frac{1}{2}$ cup stone-ground breadcrumbs
$\frac{1}{2}$ medium white onion, chopped	$\frac{1}{2}$ cup Parmesan cheese
1 TB. garlic, minced	$\frac{1}{4}$ tsp. freshly ground black pepper
1 TB. balsamic vinegar	

1. Preheat oven to 375°F.

2. Remove stems from mushrooms. Chop stems and set aside mushroom tops.

3. Heat oil in a medium skillet. Add mushroom stems to skillet with zucchini, onion, garlic, and vinegar. Sauté for about 5 to 7 minutes, until onion and zucchini start to soften. Add red peppers and heat through, about 2 minutes.

4. Remove mixture from heat and transfer to a medium bowl. Stir in basil, breadcrumbs, and cheese. Season with pepper.

5. Fill mushroom tops with vegetable mixture and bake for 15 minutes, or until mushrooms look tender and cheese is slightly melted.

TABLE TALK

Be sure to select very large mushrooms for this recipe—they'll be holding a large quantity of delectable ingredients.

Grain Side Dishes

Chapter 16

In This Chapter

- The earthy taste of whole grains
- Ways to keep inflammation from grain starches low
- Excellent gluten-free grain alternatives
- Delicious grain recipes, from traditional pilafs to creamy risottos

Whole grains provide you with high energy and filling carbohydrates. They often help folks make the transition from eating white bread and starchy boxed cereals to eating anti-inflammatory foods.

The whiter and fluffier the starch—think white bread, white rice, and large baked potatoes—the more inflammation it causes. On the other hand, the denser, chewier, and heavier the starch, the less inflammatory it is. That's why experts recommend whole grains, such as wheat berries, barley, corn, and rice.

If you have celiac disease, are gluten intolerant, or are allergic to wheat products, you need to avoid whole grains that contain gluten. This means all forms of wheat, including wheat berries, spelt, and couscous. Barley and rye also contain gluten, so don't eat those. Purchase only oatmeal products, such as steel-cut oats and old-fashioned rolled oats, that are labeled as gluten free.

You can easily change out the grains in our recipes to meet your dietary restrictions. Cooking times may vary, however.

In these 15 recipes, you'll discover many interesting and delicious ways to enjoy whole grains.

Barley Pilaf with Walnuts

Walnuts top a baked dish of barley, yams, and mushrooms flavored with parsley and thyme.

Yield:	Prep time:	Cook time:	Serving size:
6 cups	15 minutes	45 minutes	1 cup

Each serving has:				
235 calories	8.1 g total fat	1.4 g saturated fat	0 mg cholesterol	378 mg sodium
34.9 g carbohydrates	7.1 g fiber	2.7 g sugars	8.5 g protein	

1 TB. olive oil	1 cup uncooked pearl barley
8 oz. cremini mushrooms, sliced (about 3½ cups)	1 tsp. garlic, minced
¼ tsp. salt	3½ cups low-fat, low-sodium vegetable broth
5 oz. yams, cut into ½-in. cubes (about 1 cup)	2 tsp. dried parsley
½ cup green onions, diced	1 tsp. dried thyme
1 stalk celery, sliced (about ½ cup)	¼ tsp. paprika
	⅛ cup walnuts, chopped

1. Preheat oven to 400°F.

2. Heat oil in a large skillet over medium-high heat. Add mushrooms and salt, and cook, stirring often, until mushrooms begin to release their moisture, about 2 minutes.

3. Add yams, green onions, and celery, to the skillet, and continue to cook, stirring, until mushrooms are brown and yams are tender, about 4 minutes.

4. Add barley and garlic to the skillet, and stir until slightly toasted, about 1 minute. Stir in broth, parsley, thyme, and paprika.

5. Transfer mixture to an 11-cup casserole dish, cover with aluminum foil, and bake in the oven about 35 minutes until barley is tender and liquid has been absorbed. Remove foil, sprinkle with walnuts, and return to the oven. Bake, uncovered, until walnuts are toasted, about 10 minutes.

TABLE TALK

Serve this rich, savory barley side dish with meat, fish, or poultry. It's also delicious served cold or at room temperature in a lunchbox.

Quinoa Fiesta Salad

Southwestern flavor greets you with the sweet and spicy taste of black beans, jalapeño peppers, mango, and cilantro.

Yield:	Prep time:	Cook time:	Serving size:
12 cups	10 minutes	10 to 15 minutes	1 cup

Each serving has:				
300 calories	6.1 g total fat	0.9 g saturated fat	0 mg cholesterol	6.1 mg sodium
50.7 g carbohydrates	9.1 g fiber	5.4 g sugars	13 g protein	

4 cups water	1 medium red bell pepper, cored, seeded, and chopped
2 cups quinoa	1 medium orange bell pepper, cored, seeded, and chopped
¼ cup olive oil	
2 TB. lime juice	1 mango, peeled and chopped
1 TB. ground cumin	1 jalapeño pepper, seeded and chopped
¼ tsp. salt	
¼ tsp. freshly ground black pepper	3 TB. fresh cilantro, chopped
3 cups frozen corn kernels, thawed	
1 (15-oz.) can black beans, drained and rinsed	

1. In a medium saucepan, bring water to a boil. Add quinoa, cover, and reduce to a simmer. Cook for 10 to 15 minutes, until water is absorbed. Let cool.

2. Meanwhile, prepare dressing. In a jar with a screw-top lid, place oil, lime juice, cumin, salt, and pepper. Close jar and shake to blend ingredients.

3. In a large bowl, combine corn, beans, bell peppers, mango, jalapeño, and cilantro. Add quinoa, and stir to combine. Pour dressing on salad, and toss. Serve cold or at room temperature.

HEALTHY NOTE

This grain dish offers you a balanced meal with adequate protein, carbohydrates, and healthy fat.

Polenta with Italian Herbs

This side dish is flavored with the Italian herbs of parsley and basil, blended with Parmesan cheese.

Yield:	Prep time:	Cook time:	Serving size:
4 cups	15 minutes	30 minutes	1 cup

Each serving has:				
185 calories	2.7 g total fat	1.4 g saturated fat	7 mg cholesterol	295 mg sodium
33.4 g carbohydrates	1.1 g fiber	1 g sugars	6.2 g protein	

2 cups water

2 cups low-fat, low-sodium vegetable stock

1 cup polenta

$\frac{1}{3}$ cup Parmesan cheese, finely grated

$1\frac{1}{2}$ TB. fresh flat-leaf parsley, finely chopped

$1\frac{1}{2}$ TB. fresh basil, finely chopped

1. Combine water and stock in a medium pot and bring to a boil. Gradually add polenta to liquid, stirring constantly. Reduce heat and cook, stirring, about 10 minutes or until polenta thickens. Stir in cheese, parsley, and basil.

2. Spread polenta evenly into deep 8-inch-square cake pan; cool 10 minutes. Cover; refrigerate about 3 hours or until firm.

3. Turn polenta onto cutting board; trim edges. Cut into four squares, and cut each square diagonally into two triangles. Cook polenta, in batches, on a heated oiled grill or grill pan until browned on both sides.

Variation: Add 1 teaspoon minced garlic along with the cheese for a distinct Italian flavor.

TABLE TALK

You can use this polenta as a base for marinara sauce and basil-and-pine-nut pesto. Or serve as a side dish for soup, salad, meats, poultry, or eggs.

Buckwheat and Lentil Pilaf

Walnuts and apple add interest and a crunchy texture to this pilaf.

Yield:	Prep time:	Cook time:	Serving size:
4 cups	5 minutes	19 minutes	⅔ cup

Each serving has:				
220 calories	6 g total fat	0.6 g saturated fat	0 mg cholesterol	105 mg sodium
35.5 g carbohydrates	8.9 g fiber	3.4 g sugars	9 g protein	

2 tsp. olive oil

4 tsp. garlic, minced

1 cup roasted buckwheat groats

½ cup lentils

3 cups boiling water

¾ tsp. ground coriander

¼ tsp. salt

½ tsp. freshly ground black pepper

¼ cup walnuts, toasted and chopped

1 medium Granny Smith apple, cored and diced

2 tsp. walnut oil or olive oil

1. In a large skillet, heat 2 teaspoons olive oil over medium heat. Add garlic and cook until softened, about 1 minute. Stir in buckwheat grouts and lentils, and cook until buckwheat is well coated, about 3 minutes.

2. Add boiling water, coriander, salt, and pepper, and bring to a boil. Reduce to a simmer, cover, and cook until buckwheat is tender, about 15 minutes. Stir in walnuts, apple, and walnut oil.

TABLE TALK

To toast the walnuts, place in a small pan in a 350°F oven or in a small ungreased skillet over medium heat, and stir every 2 minutes until crisp and fragrant, 5 to 7 minutes.

Mushroom Pilaf with Wild Rice

Flax seeds and wild rice add crunch and flavor along with sautéed mushrooms.

Yield:	Prep time:	Cook time:	Serving size:
4 cups	10 minutes	28 minutes	⅔ cup

Each serving has:				
258 calories	5.9 g total fat	1.7 g saturated fat	5 mg cholesterol	222 mg sodium
43.9 g carbohydrates	4.8 g fiber	2.8 g sugars	10.2 g protein	

1 TB. olive oil

1 TB. butter

¾ cup yellow onion, minced

10 oz. cremini or white mushrooms, diced

¼ cup fresh parsley, snipped

½ tsp. salt

¼ tsp. freshly ground black pepper

2 TB. flax seeds

2 tsp. lemon juice

2 cups cooked wild rice

½ cup hot low-sodium chicken broth

1. Preheat oven to 450°F. Grease a 1½-quart baking dish.

2. In a large skillet, heat oil and butter over medium heat. Add onion and cook about 3 minutes, until translucent. Add mushrooms and cook for 5 minutes. Stir in parsley, salt, pepper, flax seeds, and lemon juice.

3. Stir wild rice into mushroom mixture and transfer to the baking dish. Pour broth over mixture. Cover dish and bake for 15 minutes, or until hot and bubbling. Uncover and bake for 5 more minutes.

TABLE TALK

Check out the more exotic and unusual rice blends at the grocery store. Some contain red rice, brown rice, and wild rice. You can use any of these blends in this recipe.

Brown Rice and Barley Pilaf

Enjoy this versatile side dish flavored with onion and garlic with many main course entrées and salads.

Yield:	Prep time:	Cook time:	Serving size:
3 cups	10 minutes	63 minutes	½ cup

Each serving has:				
163 calories	5 g total fat	1.7 g saturated fat	5 mg cholesterol	240 mg sodium
25.8 g carbohydrates	3.5 g fiber	0.9 g sugars	4.2 g protein	

1 TB. olive oil	½ cup barley
1 TB. butter	½ cup brown rice
1 medium yellow onion, chopped	2½ cups low-sodium chicken broth
2 tsp. garlic, minced	½ tsp. salt

1. In a medium saucepan, heat oil and butter over medium heat. Add onion, garlic, barley, and rice, and cook, stirring constantly, until onion is translucent, about 3 minutes.

2. Stir in broth and salt. Bring to a boil over high heat, and then reduce to a simmer, cover tightly, and cook until liquid has been absorbed and barley and rice are tender, about 1 hour.

HEALTHY NOTE

If you want to enrich any of the grain dishes by adding omega-3 essential fatty acids, toss in 1 to 2 tablespoons of flax seeds before baking or simmering.

Papaya Barley Salad

Blue cheese plays counterpoint to the sweetness of the papaya, pecans, and balsamic vinegar.

Yield:	Prep time:	Cook time:	Serving size:
8 cups	10 minutes	1 hour	1⅓ cups

Each serving has:				
164 calories	12.1 g total fat	1.8 g saturated fat	2 mg cholesterol	158 mg sodium
12.4 g carbohydrates	3.1 g fiber	2 g sugars	2.9 g protein	

2 cups water	2 TB. blue cheese, crumbled
¼ tsp. salt	6 cups field greens, shredded
⅓ cup barley	2 TB. balsamic vinegar
½ cup pecan pieces, toasted	2 TB. olive oil
1 small papaya, thinly sliced	

1. In a large saucepan, bring water to a boil. Add salt and barley, reduce heat to simmer, and cook until barley is tender, about 45 minutes. Drain and remove to a large salad bowl.

2. Toss warm barley with pecan pieces, papaya, and blue cheese. Add field greens and toss. Drizzle with balsamic vinegar and olive oil. Toss and serve.

TABLE TALK

In this recipe, you're making balsamic vinaigrette as you toss the salad. A rule-of-thumb recipe is to mix equal amounts of olive oil and vinegar. Additional spices are optional.

Parmesan Barley Risotto

This risotto is made from barley and Parmesan cheese and flavored with carrots and tarragon.

Yield:	Prep time:	Cook time:	Serving size:
6 cups	10 minutes	25 minutes	1 cup

Each serving has:				
288 calories	10.4 g total fat	3.7 g saturated fat	15 mg cholesterol	270 mg sodium
37.6 g carbohydrates	8.5 g fiber	1.5 g sugars	12.5 g protein	

1 cup leeks, chopped

2 TB. olive oil

1½ cups quick-cooking barley

3¾ cups hot water

1 cup Parmesan cheese, finely shredded

½ cup carrots, shredded

1 TB. fresh tarragon, snipped

1. In saucepan, sauté leeks in olive oil until softened. Add barley. Cook and stir for 1 minute. Add water, ½ cup at a time, stirring in each addition until liquid is absorbed and creamy, about 25 minutes.

2. Remove saucepan from heat. Stir in cheese, carrots, and tarragon. Serve immediately.

TABLE TALK

The secret to obtaining a creamy risotto is to continue stirring as the barley cooks.

Barley Salad with Corn and Olives

Green olives provide tang to this salad composed with corn and red bell pepper.

Yield:	Prep time:	Cook time:	Serving size:
6 cups	10 minutes	60 minutes	¾ cup

Each serving has:				
174 calories	6.8 g total fat	1 g saturated fat	0 mg cholesterol	243 mg sodium
25.3 g carbohydrates	5.5 g fiber	2.1 g sugars	4.5 g protein	

1 cup regular barley

2 cups low-sodium chicken broth

1½ cups fresh or frozen corn kernels

1 large red bell pepper, cored, seeded, and chopped (1 cup)

½ cup red onion, chopped

1 small bunch parsley, finely snipped (½ cup)

½ cup pimiento-stuffed green olives, drained and sliced

¼ cup cider vinegar

3 TB. olive oil

½ tsp. salt

½ tsp. paprika

1. In a large saucepan, combine barley and broth. Bring to a boil and then reduce heat. Cover and simmer for 45 minutes or until barley is tender and most of the liquid is absorbed. Drain. Rinse with cold water and then drain again.

2. In a large bowl, stir together barley, corn, bell pepper, onion, parsley, and olives.

3. For dressing, in a small bowl, whisk together vinegar, olive oil, salt, and paprika. Pour dressing over vegetable mixture and toss to coat. Serve.

TABLE TALK

Barley adds great texture and chewing satisfaction to this salad.

Couscous with Garlic Shrimp

Shrimp flavored with oregano and thyme top couscous, sun-dried tomatoes, and spinach.

Yield:	Prep time:	Cook time:	Serving size:
12 cups	30 minutes	3 to 5 minutes	2 cups

Each serving has:				
334 calories	13.3 g total fat	3.8 g saturated fat	0 g trans fat	183 mg cholesterol
398 mg sodium	33.1 g carbohydrates	4.4 g fiber	0 g sugars	25 g protein

24 large fresh or frozen shrimp, peeled and deveined

1 TB. olive oil

4 tsp. garlic, minced

1 tsp. dried oregano, crushed

$\frac{1}{2}$ tsp. dried thyme, crushed

1 cup dry couscous

$1\frac{1}{4}$ cups water

1 (8-oz.) jar oil-packed sun-dried tomatoes, drained and chopped

2 TB. lemon juice

2 TB. butter, melted

1 (6-oz.) package (4 cups) fresh baby spinach

6 kalamata or ripe olives, pitted and halved

1. Place shrimp in a large resealable plastic bag. Add olive oil, garlic, oregano, and thyme. Seal and turn to coat shrimp evenly. Marinate in the refrigerator for 1 hour.

2. Meanwhile, place couscous in a medium heat-resistant bowl. Bring water to a boil, and then pour over couscous. Stir, and then cover and let sit for 5 minutes or until water is absorbed. Stir in tomatoes. Set aside.

3. In a small bowl, combine lemon juice and butter; set aside.

4. In a large skillet, cook and stir shrimp with marinade over medium heat for 3 to 5 minutes or until shrimp turn opaque.

5. To serve, arrange spinach on a serving platter or divide among 6 bowls. Spoon couscous mixture over spinach. Arrange shrimp over couscous and spoon butter mixture over all. Top with olives.

TABLE TALK

Couscous is a pasta made from whole-grain semolina wheat. It originated in Berber cuisine in North Africa.

Wheat Berries with Dried Apricots

Garbanzo beans and peas add protein to the wheat berries sweetened with apricots and cranberries.

Yield:	Prep time:	Cook time:	Serving size:
8 cups	20 minutes plus overnight soak	45 minutes	1 cup

Each serving has:				
122 calories	2.9 g total fat	0 g saturated fat	0 mg cholesterol	175 mg sodium
20.3 g carbohydrates	3.5 g fiber	4.4 g sugars	5.9 g protein	

1 cup wheat berries, rinsed and drained

3 cups water

$\frac{1}{8}$ teaspoon salt

1 (15-oz.) can garbanzo beans, rinsed and drained

1 cup frozen peas, thawed

$\frac{1}{2}$ cup dried apricots, sliced

$\frac{1}{2}$ cup dried unsweetened cranberries

1 red bell pepper, cored, seeded, and chopped

3 TB. walnut oil

1 TB. lemon juice

$\frac{1}{4}$ tsp. salt

$\frac{1}{8}$ tsp. freshly ground black pepper

1. In a medium bowl, combine wheat berries, water, and salt. Cover and refrigerate overnight.

2. Transfer wheat berries to a medium saucepan and bring to a boil. Reduce heat and simmer, covered, 45 to 60 minutes or until tender. Drain. Cool for 1 hour.

3. In a large bowl, combine wheat berries, garbanzo beans, peas, apricots, cranberries, and bell pepper.

4. In a small bowl, whisk together oil, lemon juice, salt, and pepper. Pour over wheat berry mixture. Stir to coat. Serve at once or cover and refrigerate up to 24 hours.

TABLE TALK

You can serve this dish chilled, at room temperature, or heated. To heat, place wheat berry combination in the oven at 350°F for 20 to 30 minutes. Remove from heat, and stir in the oil and lemon dressing.

Risotto with Mushrooms

Wheat berries and rice combine to make a delectable risotto with the sharp, fragrant taste of asiago cheese.

Yield:	Prep time:	Cook time:	Serving size:
8 cups	15 minutes	4½ hours	1 cup

Each serving has:				
287 calories	9.8 g total fat	5.6 g saturated fat	24 mg cholesterol	684 mg sodium
37.7 g carbohydrates	1.4 g fiber	2 g sugars	12.2 g protein	

½ cup wheat berries

1½ cups water

1¼ lb. fresh crimini mushrooms, sliced

3 (14-oz.) cans reduced-sodium chicken broth

1⅔ cups converted rice

½ cup white onion, chopped

3 tsp. garlic, minced

2 tsp. dried oregano

¼ tsp. freshly ground black pepper

4 oz. asiago cheese, finely shredded

3 TB. butter, cut up

2 TB. fresh Italian flat-leaf parsley, chopped

1. In a small saucepan, combine wheat berries and water. Bring to boiling. Reduce heat and simmer, covered, for 30 minutes. Drain.

2. Place wheat berries, mushrooms, broth, rice, onion, garlic, oregano, and pepper in a 4- or 5-quart slow cooker. Cover and cook on the low heat setting for 4 hours or until rice is tender.

3. Stir cheese and butter into rice. Turn off the cooker. Let stand, covered, 15 minutes. Stir in additional broth if risotto is too dry.

4. To serve risotto, top with parsley.

HEALTHY NOTE

Use only converted rice in this recipe. Converted rice is quite viable as a low-inflammation food because it's low-glycemic. You can use it when you need to cook up a quick batch of rice for dinner.

Wild Rice Risotto with Spinach

Wild rice, carrots, spinach, and peas combine with Parmigiano-Reggiano cheese and are topped with the flavors of onion, radishes, and tarragon.

Yield:	Prep time:	Cook time:	Serving size:
6 cups	15 minutes	35 to 45 minutes	1 cup

Each serving has:				
204 calories	7.5 g total fat	2.3 g saturated fat	7 mg cholesterol	181 mg sodium
26 g carbohydrates	3.6 g fiber	2.7 g sugars	9.4 g protein	

2 tsp. garlic, minced

2 TB. olive oil

½ cup carrot, thinly sliced

1 cup wild rice

1¾ cups water

2 cups fresh spinach leaves, coarsely chopped

1 cup frozen baby or regular peas

2 oz. Parmigiano-Reggiano cheese, shredded

⅓ cup green onions, thinly sliced

¼ cup fresh radishes, trimmed and cut into thin wedges

2 tsp. fresh tarragon, snipped

1. In a 3-quart saucepan, cook garlic in hot oil over medium heat for 30 seconds. Stir in carrots and rice. Remove from heat.

2. Meanwhile, in a medium saucepan, bring water to a boil. Reduce heat and simmer.

3. Carefully stir 1 cup of the hot water into rice mixture. Cook, stirring frequently, over medium heat until liquid is absorbed. Then add ½ cup of the broth at a time, stirring frequently, until broth is absorbed before adding more broth. Cook and stir just until rice is tender and rice kernels begin to open, 30 to 45 minutes.

4. Stir in spinach, peas, cheese, onion, radishes, and tarragon until they are heated throughout, about 5 minutes. Remove to a serving bowl. Serve immediately.

HEALTHY NOTE

The carrots, spinach, and peas add antioxidants and vegetable fiber to this yummy risotto.

Brown Rice Salad with Corn

This whole-grain salad is boosted with corn, tomatoes, and jalapeño peppers.

Yield:	Prep time:	Cook time:	Serving size:
8 cups	10 minutes	3 to 5 minutes	⅔ cup

Each serving has:				
249 calories	5.3 g total fat	0.8 g saturated fat	0 mg cholesterol	88 mg sodium
47.5 g carbohydrates	4.1 g fiber	6.7 g sugars	5.6 protein	

4 cups fresh or frozen corn

1½ cups cooked brown rice, cooled

1 pint cherry or grape tomatoes, halved

1 cup fresh arugula, torn into bite-size pieces

1 small red onion, cut into thin wedges

1 fresh jalapeño pepper, thinly sliced

2 TB. balsamic vinegar

2 TB. olive oil

¼ tsp. salt

¼ tsp. freshly ground black pepper

1. In a vegetable steamer, cook corn for 3 to 5 minutes, until al dente.

2. In a serving bowl, combine rice, tomatoes, arugula, onion, and jalapeño pepper. Top with corn.

3. Drizzle mixture with vinegar and olive oil. Sprinkle with salt and ground black pepper and toss. Serve at room temperature.

TABLE TALK

An electric rice steamer is a great way to make perfect rice every time. Use it when cooking rice, as in this recipe.

Greek Couscous with Walnuts

Walnuts accent a flavorful couscous, along with mint, oregano, and feta cheese.

Yield:	Prep time:	Cook time:	Serving size:
8 cups	10 minutes	10 minutes	1 cup

Each serving has:				
233 calories	11.9 g total fat	1.7 g saturated fat	4 mg cholesterol	258 mg sodium
24.8 g carbohydrates	5 g fiber	2.9 g sugars	8.6 g protein	

1¼ cups water

1 cup whole-wheat couscous

2 cups cherry tomatoes, halved

1 medium cucumber, coarsely chopped

1 medium green bell pepper, cored, seeded, and coarsely chopped

½ cup fresh chives, snipped

¼ cup fresh Italian flat-leaf parsley, chopped

¼ cup fresh mint, snipped

¼ cup fresh oregano, snipped

¼ cup balsamic vinegar

3 TB. olive oil

½ tsp. salt

¼ tsp. freshly ground black pepper

½ cup reduced-fat feta cheese, crumbled

½ cup walnuts, toasted and coarsely chopped

1. In a small saucepan, bring water to a boil. Stir in couscous, remove from heat, and cover for 5 minutes.

2. Meanwhile, in a large bowl, combine tomatoes, cucumber, bell pepper, chives, parsley, mint, and oregano. Fold in couscous.

3. In a small bowl, whisk together balsamic vinegar, olive oil, salt, and pepper. Pour over couscous mixture and toss to combine. Spoon into serving bowl, or cover and chill up to 24 hours. To serve, top with feta cheese and walnuts.

HEALTHY NOTE

Using reduced-fat feta cheese makes a big difference in the amount of fat in this recipe—and it tastes great.

Desserts

In This Chapter

- Delicious anti-inflammation desserts
- Ways to cook with minimal amounts of sweeteners
- Healthier dessert treats

The finale for most cookbooks is a dessert chapter, and in writing this chapter, our challenge was to give you options for special-occasion desserts. Since most desserts are based on using sugar and wheat, we honed these recipes to deliver delicious and varied tastes while using minimal amounts of those two ingredients.

Most of the recipes have no sugar, but some do. If a recipe needs a bit of sweetener, we use honey, maple syrup, or sugar. We chose not to use artificial sweeteners because they contain forms of toxins that remain untested for human consumption over the long term.

Many recipes call for nut flours that you can make in your food processor in place of wheat. As always, none of our recipes contains trans fats.

To satisfy your sweet tooth, the recipes contain such ingredients as fruit, cocoa, vanilla, nuts, some cheeses, and unsweetened fruit preserves.

We hope you enjoy them for special occasions and that your friends and family do, too.

Pumpkin Mousse

The traditional pumpkin pie seasonings of nutmeg and cinnamon are enhanced with balsamic vinegar to flavor this holiday dessert.

Yield:	Prep time:	Cook time:	Serving size:
4 cups	10 minutes	None	$\frac{2}{3}$ cup

Each serving has:				
169 calories	4.9 g total fat	3 g saturated fat	18 mg cholesterol	504 mg sodium
12.6 g carbohydrates	2.1 g fiber	6.8 g sugars	10.2 g protein	

8 oz. reduced-fat feta cheese, crumbled

½ cup low-fat plain yogurt

1 tsp. vanilla

1 TB. honey

1 (15-oz.) can 100% pure pumpkin purée

½ tsp. nutmeg

1 tsp. cinnamon

A few drops balsamic vinegar, optional

1. In a medium bowl, mix feta cheese with yogurt, vanilla, and honey.

2. Place pumpkin in a small bowl. Stir in nutmeg and cinnamon.

3. Spoon pumpkin mixture into 6 dessert bowls, dividing evenly. Top with feta cheese mixture. Add a couple drops balsamic vinegar, if desired.

TABLE TALK

This creamy pumpkin dessert only tastes rich. It's quick to make and a superb substitute for a traditional pumpkin pie, but without all the calories and fat.

Chocolate Figs

Flavorful and healthful figs are brimming with the tastes of almonds, cocoa, and cloves.

Yield:	Prep time:	Cook time:	Serving size:
12 figs	15 minutes	10 minutes	3 figs

Each serving has:			
189 calories	4.3 g total fat	0.7 g saturated fat	0 mg cholesterol 8 mg sodium
40.8 g carbohydrates	8.2 g fiber	27.6 g sugars	4.2 g protein

¼ cup almonds, toasted and chopped	12 dried figs
½ tsp. ground cloves	¼ cup unsweetened cocoa powder

1. Preheat oven to 350°F.

2. In a small bowl, combine almonds and cloves.

3. Make a slit halfway through each fig. Insert 1 teaspoon of almond mixture into slit of each fig. Close figs firmly and put on a baking sheet lined with parchment paper. Bake for 5 to 10 minutes.

4. As soon as figs start to brown, remove from the oven and, while still hot, roll them in cocoa powder. Serve warm or at room temperature.

TABLE TALK

Serve these figs after dinner with coffee and tea, or box them and give them as a healthy holiday treat. They'll stay good in the refrigerator for one week.

Watermelon with Basil

Watermelon cubes are flavored with basil and vanilla, and topped with chocolate chips and a splash of balsamic vinegar.

Yield:	Prep time:	Cook time:	Serving size:
4 cups	15 minutes plus 30 minutes chill time	None	1 cup

Each serving has:				
68 calories	1.3 g total fat	0.8 g saturated fat	1 mg cholesterol	5 mg sodium
13.8 g carbohydrates	0.8 g fiber	11.4 g sugars	1.2 g protein	

4 cups seedless watermelon cubes

1 tsp. vanilla extract

2 TB. fresh basil, snipped

4 tsp. chocolate chips (preferably small ones)

2 tsp. balsamic vinegar, optional

1. Place watermelon in 4 large dessert bowls. Sprinkle with vanilla and basil. Chill for 30 minutes.

2. Sprinkle the dessert bowls with chocolate chips and a dash of balsamic vinegar, if using.

TABLE TALK

The chocolate chips resemble watermelon seeds. If the small chips aren't available at your favorite grocery store, you can coarsely chop the larger ones.

Hazelnut Stuffed Peaches

The delectable flavor of fresh peaches is accented with hazelnuts and a splash of honey.

Yield:	Prep time:	Cook time:	Serving size:
12 halves	15 minutes	None	2 halves

Each serving has:				
79 calories	2.3 g total fat	0 g saturated fat	1 mg cholesterol	77 mg sodium
12.6 g carbohydrates	1.8 g fiber	10.3 g sugars	3.4 g protein	

3 oz. low-fat cream cheese

2 tsp. honey

¼ cup hazelnuts, toasted and chopped

6 peaches, halved and pitted

Dash cinnamon

1. In a food processor, combine cream cheese, honey, and hazelnuts. Process until combined.

2. Equally divide cream cheese mixture among the 12 peach halves, placing in the depressions from the pits.

3. Serve chilled, topping each with a dash of cinnamon.

Variation: This recipe can be modified by using plums or nectarines in place of the peaches, and by substituting pecans, walnuts, or pine nuts in place of the hazelnuts.

TABLE TALK

Making desserts with fruit, as in these stuffed peaches, counts as one fruit serving while satisfying a person's desire for something sweet at the end of a meal.

Chocolate Macaroons

These delectable cookies are filled with healthful coconut and flavored with chocolate and vanilla.

Yield:	Prep time:	Cook time:	Serving size:
24 cookies	10 minutes	14 to 15 minutes	1 cookie

Each serving has:				
62 calories	3.1 g total fat	2.5 g saturated fat	1 mg cholesterol	24 mg sodium
7.5 g carbohydrates	0.8 g fiber	6.4 g sugars	1.1 g protein	

3 oz. dark chocolate, chopped

1¾ cups unsweetened coconut, shredded

½ cup granulated sugar

3 TB. unsweetened cocoa powder

⅛ tsp. salt

½ cup egg whites (about 4 egg whites)

1 tsp. vanilla extract

1. Preheat oven to 350°F.

2. Line a large baking sheet with parchment paper. In a small microwave-safe bowl, melt chocolate in the microwave on high for 45 seconds. Stir and continue to microwave in 15-second intervals, stirring after each, until melted. Set aside to cool.

3. In a large bowl, mix together coconut, sugar, cocoa powder, and salt. Stir in melted chocolate until just combined.

4. In a small bowl, whisk egg whites with vanilla extract until mixture forms stiff peaks, but isn't dry. Add to coconut mixture and stir until well blended.

5. Make each cookie using one level tablespoonful of batter. Make 24 cookies. Bake for 14 to 15 minutes, until outer layers are firm, bottoms are lightly browned, and centers remain soft. Remove from oven and let cool on baking sheet for 5 minutes.

TABLE TALK

Use the darkest chocolate you can find, between 60 and 85 percent. This makes the chocolate taste strong. You can now find 63 percent chocolate chips at the grocery store, so you may want to use them. Not to worry about the sugar content—each cookie contains only 1 teaspoon of sugar.

Flavored Hot Cocoa

Your choice of tea adds fragrance and flavor to hot cocoa.

Yield:	Prep time:	Cook time:	Serving size:
1 mug	10 minutes	None	1 mug

Each serving has:				
71 calories	0.7 g total fat	0 g saturated fat	1 mg cholesterol	15 mg sodium
16.9 g carbohydrates	1.8 g fiber	14.1 g sugars	1.9 g protein	

1 cup boiling water

1 teabag, chocolate-flavored tea or your choice

1 TB. unsweetened cocoa powder

1 TB. granulated sugar

2 TB. nonfat dry, powdered milk

Optional: orange peel, ground cloves, cardamom, vanilla extract, almond extract, peppermint extract, nutmeg, chili powder, cinnamon

1. In a mug, pour boiling water over teabag. Let steep for 5 to 10 minutes, depending on your preference for strong tea. Remove teabag.

2. Stir in cocoa powder, sugar, and powdered milk.

3. Based on the flavors in your tea, add any or a combination of the following flavors: orange peel, ground cloves, cardamom, vanilla extract, almond extract, peppermint extract, nutmeg, chili powder, cinnamon, or another you'd enjoy.

TABLE TALK

Yes, tea and cocoa pair together well. Each complements the other in taste. To choose the flavor of your cocoa, you can draw on the many choices of flavored chocolate bars that are widely available.

Honey-Glazed Pears with Blueberries

Blueberries, vanilla, and lemon add flavor to honey-glazed pears.

Yield:	Prep time:	Cook time:	Serving size:
8 pear halves	10 minutes	5 minutes	1 half-pear

Each serving has:				
73 calories	0.1 g total fat	0 g saturated fat	0 mg cholesterol	1 mg sodium
19.1 g carbohydrates	3.4 g fiber	12.9 g sugars	0.5 g protein	

4 ripe Asian pears, halved, cored, and seeded	1 tsp. lemon zest, finely grated
1 TB. honey	1 tsp. pure vanilla extract
	¼ cup fresh blueberries

1. Arrange an oven rack about 5 inches from the broiler and heat the broiler on high. Line a rimmed baking sheet with foil.

2. Arrange pear halves, cut sides up, on the prepared baking sheet.

3. In a small ramekin, stir together honey, lemon zest, and vanilla extract. Spoon blueberries equally into each pear half. Spoon honey mixture on top of blueberries.

4. Broil pears, rotating the pan once, until bubbling and caramelized, about 5 minutes. Serve warm.

Variation: You can substitute Bosc or Bartlett pears for the Asian pears in this recipe. All of them complement the taste of the blueberries and go well with vanilla.

TABLE TALK

Select pears that are barely ripe. If they aren't ripe enough, your dessert with be crunchy, if they're overly ripe, the dessert could turn into mush.

Grilled Mint Julep Pineapple

Grilling brings out the sweetness of the pineapple, while the mint-infused bourbon adds sparkle and fragrance.

Yield:	Prep time:	Cook time:	Serving size:
8 spears	10 minutes	4 minutes	2 spears

Each serving has:				
78 calories	0.2 g total fat	0 g saturated fat	0 mg cholesterol	3 mg sodium
16 g carbohydrates	2 g fiber	11.6 g sugars	0.8 g protein	

¼ cup thinly sliced fresh mint leaves, plus 4 sprigs for garnish

2 TB. bourbon
1 fresh whole pineapple

1. Heat the grill to medium.

2. Put mint and bourbon in a small bowl. Stir, pressing against the mint to release its flavor and fragrance.

3. Using a serrated knife, remove the top and a thin slice of the base from pineapple. Stand pineapple on one end and cut away all skin and brown spots; then cut the flesh into quarters lengthwise. Turn each pineapple quarter on a flat side and cut out most of the core. Cut each quarter in half lengthwise, to make 8 long spears.

4. Put pineapple spears on the hot grill. Cook, turning, until they're caramelized on each side, about 4 minutes.

5. Arrange pineapple spears on dessert plates and drizzle with bourbon mint sauce. Garnish with mint sprigs and serve immediately.

TABLE TALK

Pineapple seems to become sweeter when it's grilled, but don't worry—these are quite low in calories.

Citrus Pomegranate Terrine

This visually beautiful terrine holds delicious tangy orange and grapefruit sections along with pomegranate seeds.

Yield:	Prep time:	Cook time:	Serving size:
8 slices	20 minutes plus 4 hours chill time	None	1 slice

Each serving has:				
120 calories	0.3 g total fat	0 g saturated fat	0 mg cholesterol	2 mg sodium
27.2 g carbohydrates	3.3 g fiber	23.3 g sugars	3.7 g protein	

¾ cup fresh grapefruit juice

2 envelopes unflavored gelatin

1 cup fresh orange juice

2 (15-oz.) cans water-packed grapefruit sections, drained

2 (15-oz.) cans water-packed orange sections, drained

¼ cup pomegranate seeds

1. Pour grapefruit juice into a small, heatproof bowl and sprinkle gelatin on top. Let sit until gelatin is moist, about 3 minutes. Microwave until gelatin is dissolved and liquid is clear, 30 to 90 seconds. Add orange juice. Set aside to cool slightly, about 10 minutes.

2. In a medium bowl, place grapefruit and orange sections. Add pomegranate seeds and gently toss to combine. Pile mixture evenly into a 4½×8¼-inch loaf pan, leaving behind any extra juices. Slowly pour cooled gelatin liquid over fruit sections. Tap the loaf pan gently on the counter to release any air bubbles. Refrigerate until the top is set, and then cover the loaf pan with plastic cling wrap. Refrigerate until firm, about 4 hours, or for up to 2 days.

3. To serve, run a small knife between the gelatin and the pan, and dip the bottom of the pan into warm water for about 1 minute. Place a flat plate on top of the loaf pan. Invert and shake gently to loosen the terrine. Cut into 1-inch slices.

TABLE TALK

This is a "wow, look at me" dessert. Slice it at the table so everyone can enjoy the visual experience as well as the eating.

Blackberry Cream Parfaits

The mascarpone cheese adds a rich flavor to the blackberries, enhanced with maple syrup and walnuts.

Yield:	Prep time:	Cook time:	Serving size:
4 parfaits	10 minutes	None	1 parfait

Each serving has:				
220 calories	11.7 g total fat	4.2 g saturated fat	29 mg cholesterol	72 mg sodium
21.2 g carbohydrates	8.6 g fiber	12.2 g sugars	11.5 g protein	

⅔ cup mascarpone	2 pints blackberries
½ cup low-fat ricotta cheese	¼ cup toasted walnuts, chopped
1 TB. pure maple syrup	

1. Put mascarpone, ricotta, and maple syrup in a small bowl and stir until blended.

2. Arrange cream mixture and blackberries in parfait glasses: place some cream in the glasses, top with blackberries, and top with more cream. Add another layer of blackberries, and top with cream. Sprinkle walnuts over the top layer of cream.

Variation: Substitute your favorite berries for the blackberries. Choose from raspberries, blueberries, strawberries, and cherries.

TABLE TALK

Mascarpone is an Italian cheese made from cow's milk that's enriched with cream. By blending it with the low-fat ricotta in this recipe, you can enjoy the taste and mouthfeel of the mascarpone as you continue to eat healthfully.

Walnut Almond Drops

Toasted walnuts top these cookies flavored with almond paste.

Yield:	Prep time:	Cook time:	Serving size:
15 cookies	10 minutes	16 to 18 minutes	1 cookie

Each serving has:				
92 calories	6.5 g total fat	0.5 g saturated fat	0 mg cholesterol	16 mg sodium
7 g carbohydrates	1 g fiber	4.3 g sugars	2.7 g protein	

⅔ cup almond paste, firmly packed
  and cut into pieces

2 graham crackers

1 egg white

1 TB. flax seeds

⅔ cup walnuts, chopped

1. Put almond paste and graham crackers in a food processor. Process until fine crumbs form, about 30 seconds. Add egg white and flax seeds, and process until well blended and smooth. Refrigerate dough (still in the bowl) while the oven heats.

2. Heat oven to 350°F. Line 1 large cookie sheet with a nonstick liner. Put walnuts in a small ramekin.

3. Using a mini ice cream scoop, shape dough into 1-inch balls. Dip the top half of each ball into walnuts. Arrange, walnut sides up, on the prepared cookie sheet, about 1 inch apart.

4. Bake until puffed, slightly cracked, and golden brown, 16 to 18 minutes. Let cookies sit for 5 minutes, and then transfer to a rack to cool completely. Serve immediately, or cover and store at room temperature for up to 3 days.

HEALTHY NOTE

Each cookie is rich in omega-3 fatty acids from the flax seeds and walnuts.

Oatmeal Pecan Crisps

Cinnamon brings fragrance and flavor to these oatmeal gems.

Yield:	Prep time:	Cook time:	Serving size:
8 cookies	10 minutes	12 to 14 minutes	1 cookie

Each serving has:				
104 calories	6 g total fat	2.1 g saturated fat	8 mg cholesterol	29 mg sodium
11 g carbohydrates	1.3 g fiber	4.8 g sugars	2.1 g protein	

2 TB. butter, melted	1 egg white, slightly beaten
¼ cup brown sugar, firmly packed	¾ cup old-fashioned rolled oats
¼ tsp. ground cinnamon	¼ cup pecans, chopped

1. Heat oven to 350°F. Line 1 cookie sheet with a nonstick liner or parchment paper.

2. Put butter in a medium bowl. Add brown sugar, cinnamon, and egg white. Stir until well blended. Add oats and pecans. Mixture will be crumbly.

3. Make 8 equal-size balls, scooping up dough and pressing firmly together. Flatten each cookie into a 2-inch round and place on the cookie sheet about 1½ inches apart.

4. Bake until cookies are golden brown, 12 to 14 minutes. Remove from oven and let sit on the cookie sheet for 5 minutes. Transfer to a rack to cool.

TABLE TALK

Parchment paper is a wonderful baking tool. It is uncoated paper that you can use to line baking sheets for cookies, cakes, and french fries.

Crunchy Almond Butter Drops

Almond butter adds flavor to this homestyle cookie.

Yield:	Prep time:	Cook time:	Serving size:
20 cookies	10 minutes	12 to 14 minutes	1 cookie

Each serving has:				
114 calories	6.9 g total fat	2.1 g saturated fat	15 mg cholesterol	19 mg sodium
10.1 g carbohydrates	1.1 g fiber	7.6 g sugars	3.5 g protein	

¾ cup almond butter

3 TB. butter, at room temperature

⅔ cup granulated sugar

1 large egg

¼ cup garbanzo bean flour

1. Heat oven to 350°F. Line 2 large cookie sheets with nonstick liners or parchment paper.

2. Put almond butter, butter, and sugar in a medium bowl. Beat with an electric mixer on low speed until blended, about 1 minute.

3. Add egg. Beat on medium-low speed until just blended, about 1 minute. Add garbanzo bean flour and beat until smooth.

4. Drop dough 1 tablespoon at a time onto the prepared cookie sheet about 1½ inches apart. Bake until browned around the edges, 12 to 14 minutes.

HEALTHY NOTE

Garbanzo bean flour is widely available at health-food stores and health-food sections of grocery stores. It adds protein and fiber and has a bland taste, making it suitable for desserts.

Walnut Pastry Wheels

This walnut pastry is flavored with cherry jam.

Yield:	Prep time:	Cook time:	Serving size:
16 wheels	20 minutes	23 to 25 minutes	2 wheels

Each serving has:				
105 calories	6.9 g total fat	0.8 g saturated fat	0 mg cholesterol	15 mg sodium
9.7 g carbohydrates	0.6 g fiber	5.8 g sugars	2.3 g protein	

1 frozen puff pastry sheet, thawed

½ cup confectioners' sugar

2 TB. 100% fruit cherry jam

½ cup walnuts, finely chopped

1. Place a large piece of plastic wrap on your work area. Using a rolling pin, roll out puff pastry on the plastic into a 10×13-inch rectangle. Sprinkle the top and bottom often and generously with confectioners' sugar to prevent sticking (you won't use it all).

2. Using a spatula, spread jam evenly over dough to within ¼ inch of the edges. Sprinkle with walnuts.

3. Cut dough in half lengthwise (you'll have two 5×13-inch rectangles). Starting on one long side and using the plastic as a guide, roll up dough jellyroll style. Pinch the seam to the roll so it sticks together. Repeat with remaining dough. Wrap rolls and refrigerate until firm.

4. Heat oven to 375°F. Line 1 large cookie sheet with nonstick liner or parchment paper.

5. Arrange rolls, seam sides down, on a cutting board and cut into 1½-inch slices. Arrange slices on the cookie sheet about 1 inch apart. Bake until deep golden brown, 23 to 25 minutes. Set on a rack to cool completely. Serve immediately, or cover and store at room temperature. Store in an airtight container at room temperature for 1 week. These will stay fresh for 1 month when frozen in an airtight container.

TABLE TALK

The nutritional calculations for this recipe are adjusted, figuring that you'll actually incorporate about ¼ cup confectioners' sugar into the puff pastry.

Cocoa Walnuts

The flavor of walnuts is boosted with cocoa and a dash of cayenne.

Yield:	Prep time:	Cook time:	Serving size:
6 cups	10 minutes	20 minutes	¼ cup

Each serving has:				
178 calories	15.4 g total fat	0.9 g saturated fat	0 mg cholesterol	53 mg sodium
6.9 g carbohydrates	1.9 g fiber	4.5 g sugars	6.5 g protein	

1 egg white	1 TB. unsweetened cocoa powder
1 tsp. water	1 tsp. salt
5 cups walnut halves	½ tsp. cayenne
½ cup granulated sugar	

1. Preheat oven to 325°F. Line a 15×10×1-inch baking pan with parchment paper.

2. In a large bowl, beat together egg white and water. Add walnuts and toss to coat.

3. In a small bowl, combine sugar, cocoa powder, salt, and cayenne. Sprinkle sugar mixture over nuts. Toss to coat.

4. Spread nuts in prepared baking pan. Bake for 20 minutes. Remove parchment paper and nuts to a rack to cool. Break into pieces. Store in an airtight container for up to 2 weeks at room temperature, or freeze for later use.

HEALTHY NOTE

Walnuts give you an omega-3 boost to your food intake and are toasty delicious in this recipe.

al dente Italian for "against the teeth." this term refers to pasta or rice that's neither soft nor hard, but just slightly firm against the teeth.

allspice A spice named for its flavor, which echoes of several spices (cinnamon, cloves, nutmeg), used in many desserts and in rich marinades and stews.

antipasto A classic Italian-style appetizer that includes an assortment of meats, cheeses, and vegetables, such as prosciutto, capicolla, mozzarella, mushrooms, and olives.

artichoke heart The center part of the artichoke flower, often found canned in grocery stores.

arugula A spicy-peppery green with leaves that resemble a dandelion and have a distinctive and sharp flavor.

bake To cook in a dry oven. Dry-heat cooking often results in a crisping of the exterior of the food being cooked. Moist-heat cooking, through methods such as steaming and poaching, brings a much different, moist quality to the food.

baking powder A dry ingredient used to increase volume and lighten or leaven baked goods.

balsamic vinegar Vinegar produced primarily in Italy from a specific type of grape and aged in wood barrels. It's heavier, darker, and sweeter than most vinegars.

basil A flavorful, almost sweet, resinous herb delicious with tomatoes and used in all kinds of Italian- or Mediterranean-style dishes.

baste To keep foods moist during cooking by spooning, brushing, or drizzling with a liquid.

beat To quickly mix substances.

blanch To place a food in boiling water for about 1 minute or less to partially cook the exterior, and then submerge in or rinse with cool water to halt the cooking.

blend   To completely mix something, usually with a blender or food processor—slower than beating.

body burden   The total accumulation of all the toxins stored in your body over your lifetime. Builds up over years and adds to your inflammation levels. The toxins can include mercury, lead, air pollution particulates, secondhand (or firsthand) smoke, bisphenyl A (BPA), volatile plastic fumes, and the phthalates in perfumes and fragrances.

boil   To heat a liquid to the point at which water is forced to turn into steam, causing the liquid to bubble. To boil something is to insert it into boiling water. A rapid boil occurs when a lot of bubbles form on the surface of the liquid.

bok choy   A member of the cabbage family, with thick stems, crisp texture, and fresh flavor. It's perfect for stir-frying.

bouillon   Dried essence of stock from chicken, beef, vegetables, or other ingredients. It's a popular starting ingredient for soups because it adds flavor (and often a lot of salt).

braise   To cook with the introduction of some liquid, usually over an extended period of time.

brine   A highly salted, often seasoned liquid used to flavor and preserve foods. To brine a food is to soak, or preserve, it by submerging it in brine. The salt in the brine penetrates the fibers of the meat and makes it moist and tender.

broil   To cook in a dry oven under the overhead high-heat element.

broth   *See* stock.

brown   To cook in a skillet, turning, until the food's surface is seared and brown in color, to lock in the juices.

brown rice   A whole-grain rice, including the germ, with a characteristic pale brown or tan color. It's more nutritious and flavorful than white rice.

bruschetta (or **crostini**)   Slices of toasted or grilled bread with garlic and olive oil, often with other toppings.

bulgur   A wheat kernel that's been steamed, dried, and crushed, and is sold in fine and coarse textures.

caper   The flavorful buds of a Mediterranean plant, ranging in size from *nonpareil* (about the size of a small pea) to larger, grape-size caper berries produced in Spain.

caramelize To cook sugar over low heat until it develops a sweet caramel flavor, or to cook vegetables (especially onions) or meat in butter or oil over low heat until they soften, sweeten, and develop a caramel color.

caraway A distinctive spicy seed used for bread, pork, cheese, and cabbage dishes. It's known to reduce stomach upset, which is why it's often paired with foods like sauerkraut.

cardamom An intense, sweet-smelling spice used in baking and coffee. Common in Indian cooking.

carob A tropical tree that produces long pods from which the dried, baked, and powdered flesh—carob powder—is used in baking. The flavor is sweet and reminiscent of chocolate.

cayenne A fiery spice made from hot chile peppers, especially the cayenne chile, a slender, red, and very hot pepper.

chickpea (or **garbanzo bean**) A yellow-gold, roundish bean used as the base ingredient in hummus. Chickpeas are high in fiber and low in fat.

chile (or **chili**) Any one of many different "hot" peppers, ranging in intensity from the relatively mild ancho pepper to the blisteringly hot habanero.

chili powder A warm, rich seasoning blend that includes chili pepper, cumin, garlic, and oregano.

Chinese five-spice powder A pungent mixture of equal parts cinnamon, cloves, fennel seed, anise, and Szechuan peppercorns.

chive A member of the onion family. Chives grow in bunches of long leaves that resemble tall grass or the green tops of onions and offer a light onion flavor.

chop To cut into pieces, usually qualified by an adverb such as "*coarsely* chopped" or by a size measurement such as "chopped into $1/2$-inch pieces."

chutney A thick condiment often served with Indian curries made with fruits and/or vegetables with vinegar, sugar, and spices.

cider vinegar A vinegar produced from apple cider, popular in North America.

cilantro A member of the parsley family used in Mexican dishes (especially salsa) and some Asian dishes. Use in moderation because the flavor can overwhelm. The seed of the cilantro plant is the spice coriander.

cinnamon A rich, aromatic spice commonly used in baking or desserts. Cinnamon can also be used for delicious and interesting entrées.

clove   A sweet, strong, almost wintergreen-flavor spice used in baking.

compote   A chilled dish of fresh or dried fruit that's slowly cooked in a sugary syrup made of liquid and spices.

coriander   A rich, warm, spicy seed used in all types of recipes, from African to South American, from entrées to desserts.

cornstarch   A thickener used in baking and food processing. It's the refined starch of the endosperm of the corn kernel and is often mixed with cold liquid to make into a paste before adding to a recipe, to avoid clumps.

couscous   Granular semolina (durum wheat) that's cooked and used in many Mediterranean and North African dishes.

cream   To beat a fat such as butter, often with another ingredient, such as sugar, to soften and aerate a batter.

crimini mushroom   A relative of the white button mushroom that's brown in color and has a richer flavor. The larger, fully grown version is the portobello. *See also* portobello mushroom.

crudité   Fresh vegetables served as an appetizer, often all together on one tray.

cumin   A fiery, smoky-tasting spice popular in Middle Eastern and Indian dishes. Cumin is a seed; ground cumin seed is the most common form used in cooking.

curry   Rich, spicy, Indian-style sauces and the dishes prepared with them. A curry uses curry powder as its base seasoning.

curry powder   A ground blend of rich and flavorful spices used as a basis for curry and many other Indian-influenced dishes. Common ingredients include hot pepper, nutmeg, cumin, cinnamon, pepper, and turmeric. Some curry can also be found in paste form.

custard   A cooked mixture of eggs and milk, popular as a base for desserts.

dash   A few drops, usually of a liquid, released by a quick shake.

deglaze   To scrape up bits of meat and seasoning left in a pan or skillet after cooking. Usually this is done by adding a liquid such as wine or broth and creating a flavorful stock that can be used to create sauces.

devein   To remove the dark vein from the back of a large shrimp with a sharp knife.

dice   To cut into small cubes about $\frac{1}{4}$-inch square.

Dijon mustard   A hearty, spicy mustard made in the style of the Dijon region of France.

dill   An herb perfect for eggs, salmon, cheese dishes, and, of course, vegetables (pickles!).

dredge   To coat a piece of food on all sides with a dry substance such as flour or cornmeal.

drizzle   To lightly sprinkle drops of a liquid over food, often as the finishing touch to a dish.

edamame   Fresh, plump, pale green soybeans, similar in appearance to lima beans, often served steamed and either shelled or still in their protective pods.

endive   A green that resembles a small, elongated, tightly packed head of romaine lettuce. The thick, crunchy leaves can be broken off and used with dips and spreads.

entrée   The main dish in a meal.

extra-virgin olive oil   *See* olive oil.

extract   A concentrated flavoring derived from foods or plants through evaporation or distillation that imparts a powerful flavor without altering the volume or texture of a dish.

fennel   In seed form, a fragrant, licorice-tasting herb. The bulbs have a mild flavor and a celerylike crunch and are used as a vegetable in salads or cooked recipes.

flour   Grains ground into a meal. Wheat is perhaps the most common flour, but oats, rye, buckwheat, soybeans, and chickpeas can also be used.

fold   To combine a dense and light mixture with a circular action from the middle of the bowl.

frittata   A skillet-cooked mixture of eggs and other ingredients that's not stirred, but is cooked slowly and then either flipped or finished under the broiler.

fry   *See* sauté.

garlic   A member of the onion family, a pungent and flavorful vegetable used in many savory dishes. A garlic bulb contains multiple cloves. Each clove, when chopped, provides about 1 teaspoon garlic.

ginger   A flavorful root available fresh or dried and ground that adds a pungent, sweet, and spicy quality to a dish.

Greek yogurt   A strained yogurt that's a good natural source of protein, calcium, and probiotics. Greek yogurt averages 40 percent more protein per ounce than traditional yogurt.

herbes de Provence   A seasoning mix of basil, fennel, marjoram, rosemary, sage, and thyme, common in the south of France.

horseradish   A sharp, spicy root that forms the flavor base in condiments such as cocktail sauce and sharp mustards. Prepared horseradish contains vinegar and oil, among other ingredients. Use pure horseradish much more sparingly than the prepared version.

hummus   A thick, Middle Eastern spread made of puréed chickpeas, lemon juice, olive oil, garlic, and often tahini.

Italian seasoning   A blend of dried herbs, including basil, oregano, rosemary, and thyme.

jicama   A juicy, crunchy, sweet, large, round Central American vegetable. If you can't find jicama, try substituting sliced water chestnuts.

julienne   A French word meaning "to slice into very thin pieces."

kalamata olive   Traditionally from Greece, a medium-small, long black olive with a rich, smoky flavor.

lentil   A tiny lens-shape pulse used in European, Middle Eastern, and Indian cuisines.

leukocyte   A white blood cell that helps defend the body from disease and the results of injuries. Leukocytes are produced in the bone marrow.

marinate   To soak meat, seafood, or another food in a seasoned sauce, a marinade, that's high in acid content. The acids break down the muscle of the meat, making it tender and adding flavor.

marjoram   A sweet herb, cousin of and similar to oregano. Popular in Greek, Spanish, and Italian dishes.

meld   To allow flavors to blend and spread over time. Melding is often why recipes call for overnight refrigeration and is also why some dishes taste better as leftovers.

mesclun   Mixed salad greens, usually containing lettuce and other assorted greens such as arugula, cress, and endive.

millet   A tiny, round, yellow-colored, nutty-flavored grain, often used as a replacement for couscous.

mince   To cut into very small pieces, smaller than diced—about $\frac{1}{8}$ inch or smaller.

miso   A fermented, flavorful soybean paste, key in many Japanese dishes.

nutmeg   A sweet, fragrant, musky spice used primarily in baking.

olive   The fruit of the olive tree, commonly grown on all sides of the Mediterranean. Black olives are also called ripe olives. Green olives are immature, although they're also widely eaten. *See also* kalamata olive.

olive oil   A fragrant liquid produced by crushing or pressing olives. Extra-virgin olive oil—the most flavorful and highest quality—is produced from the first pressing of a batch of olives; oil is also produced from later pressings.

oregano   A fragrant, slightly astringent herb used in Greek, Spanish, and Italian dishes.

oxidation   The browning of fruit flesh that happens over time and with exposure to air. Minimize oxidation by rubbing the cut surfaces with lemon juice.

paprika   A rich, red, warm, earthy spice that lends a rich red color to many dishes.

parboil   To partially cook in boiling water or broth.

parsley   A fresh-tasting green, leafy herb, often used as a garnish.

pâté   A savory loaf that contains meats, poultry, or seafood; spices; and often a lot of fat. It's served cold and spread or sliced on crusty bread or crackers.

pesto   A thick spread or sauce usually made with fresh basil leaves, garlic, olive oil, pine nuts, and Parmesan cheese. Other ingredients can be added, such as sun-dried tomatoes or walnuts.

pilaf   A rice dish in which the rice is browned in butter or oil and then cooked in a flavorful liquid such as a broth, often with the addition of meats or vegetables. The rice absorbs the broth, resulting in a savory dish.

pinch   An unscientific measurement for the amount of an ingredient—typically, a dry, granular substance such as an herb or seasoning—that you can hold between your finger and thumb.

pine nut   A nut that's rich (high in fat), flavorful, and a bit pine-y. Pine nuts are a traditional ingredient in pesto and add a hearty crunch to many other recipes.

poach   To cook a food in simmering liquid such as water, wine, or broth.

polenta   A mush made from cornmeal that can be eaten hot with butter or cooked until firm and cut into squares.

porcini mushroom   A rich and flavorful mushroom used in rice and Italian-style dishes.

portobello mushroom   A mature and larger form of the smaller crimini mushroom. Brown, chewy, and flavorful, portobellos are often served as whole caps, grilled, or as thin sautéed slices. *See also* crimini mushrooms.

prosciutto   A dry, salt-cured ham that originated in Italy.

purée   To reduce a food to a thick, creamy texture, typically using a blender or food processor.

quinoa   A nutty-flavored grain that's extremely high in protein and calcium.

reduce   To boil or simmer a broth or sauce to remove some of the water content, resulting in more concentrated flavor and color.

reserve   To hold a specified ingredient for another use later in the recipe.

rice vinegar   Vinegar produced from fermented rice or rice wine, popular in Asian-style dishes. (It's not the same thing as rice wine vinegar.)

risotto   A popular Italian rice dish made by browning arborio rice in butter or oil and then slowly adding liquid to cook the rice, resulting in a creamy texture.

roast   To cook something uncovered in an oven, usually without additional liquid.

rosemary   A pungent, sweet herb used with chicken, pork, fish, and especially lamb. A little goes a long way.

roux   A mixture of butter or another fat and flour used to thicken sauces and soups.

saffron   An expensive spice made from the stamens of crocus flowers. Saffron lends a dramatic yellow color and distinctive flavor to a dish. Use only tiny amounts.

sage   An herb with a musty yet fruity, lemon-rind scent and "sunny" flavor.

sauté   To pan-cook over lower heat than what's used for frying.

savory   A popular herb with a fresh, woody taste. Can also describe the flavor of food.

sear   To quickly brown the exterior of a food, especially meat, over high heat.

sesame oil   An oil made from pressing sesame seeds. It's tasteless if clear and aromatic and flavorful if brown.

shallot   A member of the onion family that grows in a bulb, somewhat like garlic, but with a milder onion flavor. When a recipe calls for shallot, use the entire bulb.

shellfish   A broad range of seafood, including clams, mussels, oysters, crabs, shrimp, and lobster.

shiitake mushroom   A large, dark brown mushroom with a hearty, meaty flavor. It can be used fresh or dried, grilled, as a component in other recipes, and as a flavoring source for broth.

simmer   To boil gently so the liquid barely bubbles.

skillet (also **frying pan**)   A generally heavy, flat-bottomed, metal pan with a handle designed to cook food over heat on a stovetop or campfire.

skim   To remove fat or other material from the top of liquid.

steam   To suspend a food over boiling water and allow the heat of the steam (water vapor) to cook the food. This quick-cooking method preserves a food's flavor and texture.

steep   To let sit in hot water, as in steeping tea in hot water for 10 minutes.

stew   To slowly cook pieces of food submerged in a liquid. Also, a dish prepared by this method.

stir-fry   To cook small pieces of food in a wok or skillet over high heat, moving and turning the food quickly to cook all sides.

stock   A flavorful broth made by cooking meats and/or vegetables with seasonings until the liquid absorbs these flavors. The liquid is strained and the solids are discarded. Stock can be eaten alone or used as a base for soups and stews.

supreme   To cut the membrane away from citrus fruit segments.

tahini   A paste made from sesame seeds, used to flavor many Middle Eastern recipes.

tamarind   A sweet, pungent, flavorful fruit used in Indian-style sauces and curries.

tapas   A Spanish term meaning "small plate" that describes individual-size appetizers and snacks served cold or warm.

tapenade   A thick, chunky spread made from savory ingredients such as olives, lemon juice, and anchovies.

tarragon   A sweet, rich-smelling herb perfect with seafood, vegetables (especially asparagus), chicken, and pork.

tempeh   An Indonesian food made by culturing and fermenting soybeans into a cake, sometimes mixed with grains or vegetables. It's high in protein and fiber.

teriyaki A Japanese-style sauce composed of soy sauce, rice wine, ginger, and sugar that works well with seafood and most meats.

thyme A minty, zesty herb.

tofu A cheeselike substance made from soybeans and soy milk.

turmeric A spicy, pungent yellow root used in many dishes, especially Indian cuisine, for color and flavor. Turmeric is the source of the yellow color in many prepared mustards.

veal Meat from a calf, generally characterized by its mild flavor and tenderness.

vegetable steamer An insert with tiny holes in the bottom, designed to fit on or in another pot to hold food to be steamed above boiling water. *See also* steam.

vinegar An acidic liquid widely used as a dressing and seasoning, often made from fermented grapes, apples, or rice. *See also* balsamic vinegar; cider vinegar; rice vinegar; white vinegar; wine vinegar.

wasabi Japanese horseradish, a fiery, pungent condiment used with many Japanese-style dishes. It's most often sold as a powder to which you add water to create a paste.

water chestnut A tuber popular in many Asian dishes. It's white, crunchy, and juicy, and holds its texture whether cool or hot.

white mushroom A button mushroom. When fresh, white mushrooms have an earthy smell and an appealing soft crunch.

white vinegar The most common type of vinegar, produced from grain.

whole grain A grain derived from the seeds of grasses, including rice, oats, rye, wheat, wild rice, quinoa, barley, buckwheat, bulgur, corn, millet, amaranth, and sorghum.

whole-wheat flour Wheat flour that contains the entire grain.

wild rice Not a rice at all, but actually a grass. It has a rich, nutty flavor and serves as a nutritious side dish.

wine vinegar Vinegar produced from red or white wine.

yeast Tiny fungi that, when mixed with water, sugar, flour, and heat, release carbon dioxide bubbles, which, in turn, cause the bread to rise.

zest Small slivers of peel, usually from a citrus fruit such as a lemon, lime, or orange.

Resources

The study of the causes of inflammation and ways to lower it is ongoing. New information is being published in medical and research journals on a regular basis. In order for you to be more effective in managing inflammation, it's important to stay up-to-date.

You can find up-to-date information on late-breaking anti-inflammation news at these websites:

arthritis.webmd.com/about-inflammation
This website offers up-to-date information on eating and other ways to reduce inflammation.

www.hsph.harvard.edu/nutritionsource/index.html
The Nutrition Source is an excellent, leading edge website maintained by the Department of Nutrition at the Harvard School of Public Health.

www.tuftshealthletter.com/?gclid=CN3O5Lig_68CFSdeTAodiAhtEw
The Tufts University Health & Nutrition Letter provides reliable, scientifically authoritative health and nutrition advice based substantially on the research conducted at the university.

To purchase specialty food items and supplements that you can't find locally, try these websites:

www.amazon.com
You'll find most ingredients that you can't find at local stores at good prices. Their free-shipping offers can save you money, too.

www.bobsredmill.com
The Bob's Red Mill website is a terrific source of whole grain and gluten-free products. The company manufactures its products in-house, even grinding whole grains at cool temperatures with a traditional stone mill.

www.gluten-free.net
The Gluten-Free Trading Company, LLC, website is an excellent source for gluten-free foods. It offers products for people following gluten-free diets, and/or suffering from celiac disease, gluten intolerance, and food allergies.

www.sunorganic.com
This online Sun Organic Farms store carries everything organic from flax to salsa.

Index

T-U